AF540808

Food and Health

FOOD AND HEALTH

By

Dr. M. Lakshmi Narasaiah

M.A., Ph.D.

Professor & Head

Department of Economics

Sri Krishnadevaraya University Post-graduate Centre

Kurnool – 518 002

Andhra Pradesh (India)

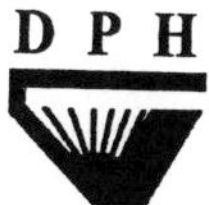

DISCOVERY PUBLISHING HOUSE PVT. LTD.

NEW DELHI-110 002

First Published – 2004

Reprinted – 2025

ISBN: 978-81-7141-828-2

Food and Health

Published by:

DISCOVERY PUBLISHING HOUSE
4383/4B, Ansari Road, Darya Ganj
New Delhi-110 002 (India)
Phone: +91-11-23279245; 23253475; 43596065
E-mail: discoverybooksindia@gmail.com
orderdphbooks@gmail.com
namitwasan9@gmail.com
web: www.discoverypublishinggroup.com

Printed at:
Infinity Imaging Systems
Delhi

Preface

The world food situation has never been better. Enough food is being produced today that, if it were evenly distributed, no one should have to go hungry. World food production is increasing faster than population growth: per capita production increased by 5 per cent during the 1980s. Real food prices are at historic lows and have been declining for some time now. Yields of major cereals have more than doubled in the past three decades. These trends have contributed to complacency in some quarters regarding the world food situation.

Yet, more than 700 million people in the developing world do not have access to sufficient food to lead healthy and productive lives. More than 180 million children are underweight. Diseases of hunger and malnutrition are widespread. The desire to satisfy food needs has, in combination with increasing population densities and inadequate agricultural intensification, led to much degradation of environmentally fragile lands, such as forests and steep hillsides.

Over the next 20-30 years, farmers and policy makers in developing countries with be challenged to provide food at affordable prices for almost 100 million more people every year—the largest annual population increase in history. Moreover, they will have to increases food production from more productive use of the land and without further degradation of natural resources: area expansion is no longer a feasible option in most of the world.

What future food security will look like depends not on exogenous factors over which we have no control but on the decisions and actions taken by the major players: households, private and public sector agencies, governments, and the international community. If we continue to act as we have in the 1980s and early 1990s, more people will suffer from food insecurity, it will be because some or all of these players failed to act in an appropriate and timely manner.

Feeding the World: Availability and Access to Food

There is enough food in the world today to feed everyone, if it were evenly distributed. Availability of daily food energy per capita in the developing countries as a whole increased by 0.7 per cent per year during the 1980s.

Twenty-five developing countries, including about half of the African countries, were unable to assure sufficient food energy (2,200 calories per person per day) for their populations at the end of the 1980s even if available food energy were evenly distributed within each country. This is down from 45 countries at the end of the 1970s.

However, available food is neither evenly distributed nor fully consumed. Availability of enough food at global, regional, or national levels does not necessarily mean that everyone is well fed. For people to be food secure—that is, to have access at all times to the food required for a healthy and productive life—there must be both availability of food and access to food. Access to food by households (and individuals) is conditioned by poverty: the poor usually lack adequate means to secure access to food.

Over 1.1 billion people in developing countries were living in poverty in 1993, more than 500 million in conditions of extreme poverty. South Asia is the home of about 50 per cent of the developing world's poor-more than 500 million people. Another 15 per cent are found in East Asia, 19 per cent in Sub-Saharan Africa, and 10 per cent in Latin America and the Caribbean. The prevalence of poverty (the proportion of each region's population that is poor) is very high-about 50 per cent—in South Asia as well as in Sub-Saharan Africa.

Today, there are more than 700 million people who do not have access to sufficient food to meet their needs for a healthy and productive life; they often go hungry adults and children also suffer from diseases associated with hunger and poverty. For almost one fifth of the total population of developing countries to be chronically hungry tarnishes the image of a world that is now considered food-secure because it produces enough food.

Great progress has been made in meeting food needs during the last 30 years. For instance, the number of underfed people declined from an estimated 976 million in 1974-76 to 786 million in late 1980s. But the problem is far from solved. Keeping up with increasing needs and demands due to population growth, income increases, and dietary changes is itself a formidable challenge.

Hunger and food insecurity have a significant effect on health and nutrition of both adults and children. They can lead to growth failure in children. About 184 million preschool children in developing countries were underweight in 1994. About 55 per cent of these underweight children were found in South Asia and another 16 per cent in Sub-Saharan Africa. The proportion of children that are underweight is higher in South Asia (almost 60 per cent), but it is also significant in Sub-Saharan Africa (30 per cent) and Southeast Asia (31 per cent). It is worrisome that the number of underweight children in Sub-Saharan Africa during the 1980s from 20 million to 28 million is particularly striking.

In addition to energy deficiencies, micro nutrient deficiencies are also widespread in the developing world. About 14 million preschool children (under the age of five years) have eye damage as a result of vitamin A deficiency. Ten million of these children are found in Southeast Asia. Between 250,000 and 500,000 preschool children go blind each year due to vitamin A deficiency, two-thirds of these children die within months of going blind. Many more children are mildly affected. Recent research has shown that even mild deficiencies can increase mortality significantly. Vitamin A deficiencies are closely linked to diet, which can be influenced by agricultural research and policy.

Dr. M. Lakshmi Narasaiah

Contents

1

Food Production

During the last 25 years, world agriculture successfully expanded food production faster than population growth. This can continue for the next 25 years and beyond, if appropriate action is taken. Although world food stocks are currently low and grain prices high, the world is not about to run out of food. We can produce enough food for future generations if we choose to do so.

The widespread food insecurity, unhealthy living conditions, and abject and absolute poverty in many developing countries are already threatening global stability. Failure to assure sustainable food security will foster the very conditions that will further destabilize and polarize the world in the years to come with tremendous consequences for all people.

The Basic Facts

Poverty is widespread in developing countries, with over 1.1 billion people living on a dollar a day or less per person. Human resource development in developing countries is lagging: 1 billion people lack access to health services, 1.3 billion do not have access to adequate sanitation systems, and one-third of primary school enrolls drop out by Grade 4. Natural resources, upon which future food production depends, are being degraded at alarming rates: almost 2 billion hectares of land have been degraded in the past 50 years: about 180 million hectares of forests have been converted to other uses during the 1980s, marine fisheries are collapsing around the world, and regional and seasonal water shortage afflict many developing countries. Improved appropriate technology is essential to increase productivity. Yet low-income food deficit developing countries are grossly underinvesting in agricultural research and many are reducing their support.

It calls for sustained action in *six* priority areas. ***First,*** we must selectively strengthen the capacity of developing country governments to perform appropriate functions such as establishing or clarifying property rights, promoting private-sector competition in agricultural markets, and maintaining appropriate macro economic environments. Predictability, transparency and continuity in policy making and enforcement must be pursued.

Investing in People

Second, we must invest more in poor people in order to enhance their productivity, health, and nutrition. It is not only unethical but economically wasteful that a large share of the World's population is malnourished, illiterate, sick, and without access to productive resources. Access to primary education, primary health care, reproductive care and family planning information, and clean water and sanitation must be assured for all people. Access by the poor to productive resources and remunerative employment must be improved. Empowerment of women must be supported.

Third, we must accelerate agricultural productivity. Agriculture is the life blood of the economy in low-income developing countries. In those countries, it provides upto three-quarters of all employment and half of all incomes. There are very strong links between agricultural productivity increases and broad-based economic growth in the rest of the economy. Agriculture is an engine of growth in low-income developing countries. National and international agricultural research systems must be mobilized to develop improved technologies focused on developing countries, and extension systems must be strengthened to disseminate the improved technologies and techniques. Low-income countries currently spend less than 0.5 per cent of the value of agricultural production on agricultural research compared to 2 per cent spent on agricultural research in middle and high-income countries. An increase of agricultural research expenditures in low-income countries to at least 1 per cent of the value of an agricultural output is urgently needed, with a longer term target of 2 per cent. National agricultural research must be supported by a vibrant international agricultural research system that undertakes research with large international benefits applicable across boundaries. Current investments in international agricultural research are grossly inadequate to provide the support needed by developing countries. It is of critical importance that agricultural research result in reduced unit-costs of production. Such cost reductions will make food economically accessible to low-income consumers, and permit producer incomes to increase. To assure relevance of research and appropriate distribution of responsibilities, interactions between public sector agricultural research systems, farmers, private enterprises, and NGOs must be strengthened.

Fourth, we must assure sustainability in agricultural production and sound management of natural resources. Farmers, local communities, and governments must be encouraged to establish and enforce systems of rights to use and manage natural resources, to improve the way water is allocated and used, to reverse land degradation where it has occurred, to reduce the use of chemical pesticides and promote integrated pest management programmes, and to implement integrated soil fertility programmes in areas with low soil fertility. Local control over natural resources must be strengthened and local capacity for organisation and management improved. Investments in less-favoured geographical areas, that is, areas with agricultural potential, irregular rainfall patterns and fragile soils must be expanded. Most poor people in developing countries reside in rural areas, and most rural poor reside in less-favoured areas. Yet, most investments, including agricultural research investments, still focus on the more-favoured areas. If we are serious about reducing poverty and protecting the natural resource base, the balance between the less-favoured and more-favoured areas must be redressed.

Fifth, we must reduce food marketing costs in low-income developing countries. The cost of bringing food from the producer to the consumer is very high in many of these countries. Efficient, effective, and low-cost agricultural markets must be developed in order to bring these costs down. Inefficient state-run firms in agricultural input markets must be phased out; investment in developing and maintaining infrastructure, especially in rural areas, must be forthcoming; policies and institutions that favour large-scale, capital-intensive market agents over small-scale, labour-intensive ones must be removed; development of small-scale credit and savings institutions must be facilitated; and technical assistance to create or strengthen small-scale, labour-intensive competitive rural enterprises must be provided.

Sixth, we must expand and realign international development assistance. Many years ago, industrialized countries had agreed to allocate at least 0.7 per cent of the gross national product (GNP) to international assistance. Most countries have not reached or do not maintain this target. Not only must the industrialized countries increase international development assistance to reach the 0.7 per cent target, but they must realign it to low-income developing countries. Also, contrary to the middle and higher-income developing countries, the poorest countries are not able to gain access to capital fıom the rapidly expanding international commercial capital market. Developing countries in turn must seek measures to diversify sources of external funding, stem capital flight; and improve the effectiveness of the aid they receive.

2

Food for the Billions

Will there be enough food to feed 8 billion people who will live on earth in 25 years' time? Surprisingly few people, at least in the industrial countries, seems to be overly concerned with this question. Whereas the world conferences on the environment, on women; human rights or social issues which were held in recent years were preceded and accompanied by intensive public debate, food does not seem to be a burning issue. Don't we have mountains of surplus food, people ask. Do we not have to pay our farmers to leave their land idle in order not to add to the glut on the world markets? And hasn't the Green Revolution ended famine even in countries like India which used to be a synonym for hungry people? So where is the problem?

The advance made in agricultural production since beginning against a background of imminent crisis are indeed remarkable. In only 20 years, yields of major crops like rice, maize and wheat in developing countries went up by 80 per cent, outpacing even the rapid increase in population. But this growth in yields has slowed down in recent years, and the aim of "food for all" is once again becoming elusive. About 800 million people still do not have access to enough food to meet their basic daily needs, nearly 200 million children suffer from protein and energy deficiencies, 88 countries—44 of them in Africa—have a deficit in food production.

Every one wants to increase food security. The definition is that "food be available at all times, that all persons have means of access to it, that it be nutritionally adequate in terms of quantity, quality and variety, and that it be acceptable within the given culture". To achieve this goal, more food must be produced—much more, because we must not only adequately feed the 5.8 billion people already on earth, but also the additional two billion who will be added to world population in the next 25 years. Critics argue that the problem is not one of production alone, but one of poverty elimination. People are not hungry because there is no food, but because they have no money to buy it, these critics say. Available resources must be better distributed to end hunger in the world.

However, even if we succeed to eliminate poverty in the next few decades—a feat which appears highly unlikely—there would still be the need to boost production, because with rising incomes people also want to eat more and better food including meat. As can already be observed in the countries of East Asia, the newly acquired wealth leads to higher consumption levels which puts additional strains on available resources are getting scarcer. Agricultural lands are being degraded at alarming speed by erosion, salinity, desertification or disappear altogether due to urban or infrastructure development. It has been estimated that 40 per cent of productive land now has diminished capacity to supply benefits to humanity due to direct human impacts of land use. Water for agricultural purposes is getting scarcer almost everywhere, and there are hardly any land reserves to be brought into production to widen the agricultural base.

In this situation, there is no alternative to increasing and improving production from the existing land area. This can only be done through research which finds the best varieties which will bring the highest yields at the lowest cost to the environment. Sustainable agriculture is the key notion—one that maintains bio-diversity, uses as little chemical inputs as possible and does not over exploit water and soil resources.

In recent years, agricultural research has been neglected-partly because of the erroneous belief that with mountains of meat and lakes of milk further production increases were not desirable. Since global grain production has stagnated and world stocks have reached an alarmingly low level last year, there has been a noticeable change of mind. To raise the awareness among governments around the world that promotion of agriculture is urgent if hunger is to be avoided in the next century.

Important work is already being done by the international agricultural research institutes which promoted the Green Revolution in the sixties and seventies and are now again in the forefront of finding solutions to the daunting task of feeding 8 billion people by the year 2020. The international Rice Research Institute (IRRI) in the Philippines, the Maize and Wheat Research Institute (CIMMYT) in Mexico or institutes like ICARDA in Syria and ICRISAT in India which work on agriculture in semi-arid and dry areas, are all seeking solutions to the problem of raising production while at the same time preserving the environment. These institutions as well as national agricultural research institutions need all the support from the public and, of course, appropriate funding, to help them accomplish their task.

The scientists are optimistic that they can develop the varieties and farming systems which will allow mankind to feed everyone on earth well into the next century. But the task is not for the scientists alone. An economic and political order must also be in place which makes it possible to eradicate poverty and allow everyone to enjoy the benefits that science can offer. Feeding the billions is, therefore not only a scientific, but first and foremost a political.

3

Food First

By the time this day is over, about 40,000 human beings—mostly children—will have died from hunger, malnutrition and related causes. Today and every day the deaths will mount, reaching an annual toll of 13 to 18 million. Few of these people will have been caught up in famine or other emergencies. Most will have suffered from a "silent" assault—the kind that seldom makes the headlines, but which claims its victims just as relentlessly.

It is intolerable that such deprivation and suffering should be allowed to exist in a world of potential food plenty. Having enough food is fundamental to all else. At the most basic level, this may entail humanitarian relief to assist people in emergency situations. In the transition from relief to development, however, we must look at systems for ensuring that societies have the capacity to produce or purchase the food they need and that it is accessible to all.

Sustainable food security fuses the goals of household food security and sustainable agriculture; it requires both. It requires looking not only at the aggregate supply of food, but also at the distribution of income and land, and at other issues: Do people have enough income to buy food? Enough land to grow their own food? Does the food distribution system deliver food where it is needed? How much food is wasted due to inadequate distribution systems? What are the implications of trends in population growth for future food needs? What is the status of women in society, and what opportunities do women have to alter rapid population growth rates? What is being done to regenerate the resource base for food production? These questions need to be asked and answered in every country.

The challenge of sustainable food security is immense, and it is growing. One billion people—20 per cent of the global population—are too poor to obtain enough food to sustain normal work. Half a billion are too poor to obtain the food needed for healthy growth of children and minimal activity of adults. Today's failure to feed people, however, may be but a prologue to a much larger failure in the future. Given likely population increases, world food output must triple over the next 50 years if the world's people are to have a nutritionally adequate diet. It will be difficult enough to achieve this expansion under favourable circumstances, and conditions may be far from favourable.

For example, according to recent estimates an area of about 1.2 billion hectares-the size of China and India combined—has experienced moderate to extreme soil deterioration since World War II as a result of human activities. Over three-fourths of that deterioration has occurred in the developing regions from causes such as overgrazing, deforestation, land clearing, unsound agricultural practices and increased soil salinity and water logging, largely from irrigation. Other environmental threats to the agricultural resource base include loss of water and genetic resources, adverse effects of pesticides and climate change, both local and global.

At the most aggregate level, the required increase in food production could be met if production grew at the historic average, that is, at the two per cent per annum rate achieved over the past half-century. But is this realistic? To produce three times more calories, all the land currently under cultivation around the world would, within 50 years, have to attain levels of productivity as high as those exhibited by the very best cropland today.

To this challenge add the possibility of diminished returns from the technological, energy and other inputs that have made agriculture so successful. Some experts believe that most of the potential for increased output of cereals—from improved plant varieties, from increased use of pesticides and fertilizers and from expanding the area under irrigation—has already been captured.

Viewed from this perspective, the goal of achieving sustainable food security in the decades ahead emerges as one of the greatest challenges humanity has ever faced. Agricultural output must be tripled, and people must have the income to buy the food they need. The erosion of the resource base must be halted and then reversed. Failure on any of these fronts will yield unprecedented human suffering.

What will it take to achieve sustainable food security? Obviously, the effort will have to be immense, both in size and complexity. Outlined below are a few simple (but no easy) steps that are absolutely essential elements of serious effort.

First, as citizens of the world, we must all come to see sustainable food security as a fundamental aspect of global peace and human security. This goes well beyond merely denouncing the use of food as a weapon.

Second, we must adopt concrete international goals, such as reducing world hunger by half over the next 10 years. We will never achieve the goal of sustainable food security unless we aim at specific milestones, and assess rigorously our progress in moving toward them.

Third, we must forge a true global partnership, a compact for sustainable food security. All countries—rich and poor-have important roles and responsibilities. There must be reciprocal responsibilities among nations, not one-way transfers.

Fourth, we must see deterioration of the agricultural resource base—terrestrial, aquatic and climatic—for what it is: a major threat to development and a major source of economic loss. Farmers are the largest group of environmental decision-makers in the world. We must ensure that they have the means to make sustainable development a reality where it counts—in the fields and fisheries.

Fifth, we must empower the people who work the land and who keep it productive. They are in the best position to decide the most appropriate ways to graft new technology onto their own traditional knowledge of seed selection, plant protection and nutrient-cycling. Special emphasis should be given to the role of women, the main providers for two-thirds of the poorest households in the developing world, as well as the producers of 60 per cent of all food grown and consumed locally.

Sixth, we must build the capacities of developing countries, both in government and in civil society. Capacity-building means empowerment for self-reliance. It means strengthening national capacities, both inside and outside government. This is essential for recognition and analysis of problems, for decision-making on courses of action and for management of systems and processes.

Seventh, not only must we build capacity in developing countries, we must also create linkages among researchers in industrial and developing countries. This will help minimize the time lag between discovery and practical utilization. In addition, analysts from various countries must work together to examine future food security issues with different scenarios of population growth, agricultural productivity, markets and trade, climate change, loss of soil and bio-diversity and, last but not least, political instability, in order to devise options for rational choices.

We know a good deal about how to rid the world of the scourge of hunger, and how to begin to move toward sustainable food security on a global basis. We know that economic growth and prosperity are necessary, though not sufficient, conditions for eradicating hunger. We also know that development efforts must encompass not only food production, but also socio-economic factors, including sustainable livelihoods for poor families, the implications of population growth rates, the status of women and girls and so forth. We also know that good words are not enough. Now more than ever before it is crucial that we marshal the political will to achieve our goals.

4

India's Food Challenge

Is India's population growing disproportionately to its food supply? Will famine once again hit millions of people? Most agriculture experts agree that a Malthusian crisis is not likely to occur in the near term. The reason; the overall food situation in India has been characterized by a large increase in regional output since the famine-ravaged 1960s.

At that time, the food situation was described as "desperate" in India. Famine had plagued India's Bihar state in the sixties. International food specialists predicted further famine because food production looked as if it would lag far behind population growth. Instead, average crop yields per acre soared, thanks to the introduction of high-yielding varieties of rice and wheat and to expanded irrigation and chemical fertilizer use. It has been called the "green revolution".

Double Role of Irrigation

The keys to the higher food production have been irrigation, the adoption of high-yielding varieties (HYVs) of foodgrains and the increased use of modern inputs such as fertilizers. Irrigation has played a double role, it has not only helped raise yields through synergistic interaction with HYVs and fertilizers, but has also contributed to considerable increases in harvested area by enabling higher cropping intensity.

Still, there are ominous clouds on Indian food horizon. In light of the region's high population growth, increased urban sprawl and rampant environmental degradation, there are signs that hunger problems could loom unless action is taken by Indian's and international development agencies.

Shrinking Base

The favourable food supply situation is likely to disappear within the next decade, due to a shrinking resource base, the earlier decades had witnessed a natural resources based growth strategy as there was adequate land and water resources for development. But this is fast disappearing due to urbanization, industrialization and ecological degradation. We should also remember that about 50 per cent of food production is from rainfed lands and a few years of drought could alter the food security which we now enjoy. The high costs of irrigation and land development, coupled with low commodity prices, are also hampering required investments and these effects will be seen in the next decade.

"By the year 2030, India will have to produce 60 per cent more rice with much fewer resources. Clearly, there will be a major challenge for scientists and policy-makers to meet the increased food demand. India's population is growing 2 per cent a year, making the challenges for regional food security a daunting task.

The solution for meeting future food demand will be breakthroughs in science and technology since yield levels have reached a plateau and are even showing signs of decline. The possibilities through biotechnology and genetic engineering are exciting and can herald another "green revolution". This is the only hope for avoiding the Malthusian dilemma.

In gauging the region's population-food squeeze, it is useful to look first at its swelling population. India—the world's second populous region contains several states with high population growth rates.

Ironic Problem

Rapid population growth dilutes and impedes economic development. An increase in the population base puts greater pressure on finite resources, both financial and natural, and, in the context, worsening of income distribution, increased poverty incidence and environmental degradation.

Moreover, there is the ironic problem, that although rapid population growth increases poverty, poverty encourages larger families through its impact on access to education and decreased prospects for child survival.

If population growth is uncontrolled, the economic and social consequences are:

- ecologial imbalance, with greater pressure on natural resources.
- increased urban crowding, with increases in demand for municipal services and infrastructure.
- a more unequal income distribution, particularly as labour supply outpaces job creation.
- signs of mass poverty, including high infant and child mortality rates, high levels of child malnutrition and hunger, poor school performance, unemployment and underemployment.

Bleak Prospects

Existing population growth rates is unsustainable, even for the relatively near future. Unless population growth rate is kept within manageable limits, the prospects for creating acceptable standards of living for low-income groups in India will be bleak.

The Indian population is growing more rapidly than ever before and will continue to do so for at least four decades. Indeed, without major technological breakthroughs and changes in patterns of consumption, even the most optimistic population growth projections are likely to be accompanied by increase in poverty, hunger and environmental degradation.

Whether we look at population, the environment or development, the next 10 years will be critical for our future, the decisions we make or don't take will widen or narrow our options for a century to come. They could decide the fate of the earth as a home for human beings.

5

Less Food Security in the South?

Combating hunger and poverty is the central point of Bread for the world's mandate. In our view, that is not so much about the quantity of food produced in the world. On the one hand, it's about its fair distribution and, on the other, the access of poor people to chances of jobs. Put another way, it's to do with access to purchasing power. In the case of agriculture, that is bound up with the question of how food is produced. Whether the technologies applied maximize employment or replace work with capital.

"Hunger Through Surplus"

The question of production, employment and distribution are tied closely to the general conditions for development. It is certainly not exclusively external economic conditions which account for hunger and under-development. Structural deficits, political conditions and wrong policies in Third World countries have become increasingly clear. However, it can still be noted that global economic framework conditions remain enormously important for the development of agriculture in the Third World.

Twenty years ago, Bread for the World publicly expounded the thesis "Hunger through surplus" and had to take much criticism for it—above all from agro-economists. But since then the contradiction between the ever-growing mountains of agricultural surpluses in the northern hemisphere and the increasing dependence on food imports of the South has become ever more apparent. Out of 120 poor developing countries, 107 today are net importers of food.

The North's surpluses of dairy products, grain, beef and sugar—which because of their production costs are exohrbitantly expensive—thrust their way on to world market and destroy local supply systems (which are cheap because of subsidies), regional trade flows, and the sales possibilities of potential Third World agro-exporters. Thus, the surpluses contribute to the situation that in many developing countries a policy of neglecting local agriculture can be continued with impurity.

Initially, the promise to work on the yawning gap between hunger and surplus in the world was upfront on WTO agenda. But the pattern of explanation was well simplified. It said that surpluses arose only in those countries which supported their agriculture positively and, in fact, partly excessively. And that agricultural deficiencies in countries of the South were caused mainly by deprivation of resources and capital. However, the concept of not only reducing neglect of agriculture in the South but also its oversubsidising in the North to a sensible degree and thereby eliminating their distortions of world markets had a great intellectual attraction. At any rate, it promised more justice in agriculture.

Subsidies Can Make Sense

To avoid misunderstandings, we have nothing against the support of agriculture in Europe. Above all not when it is done for social, ecological or agriculturally beneficial reasons.

On the contrary, agriculture's important role for food security, the sustainable handling of natural resources, the settlement of rural areas, and the social function of family farms justify a special position for it is economic life, including protection and support.

But that must not be carried so far that surpluses are produced with the help of dubious production methods and then dumped on the world market at markedly less than cost price, causing incalculable damage in the poor countries. On the otherhand, purposeful promotion of rural development is a prerequisite and model for greater self-sufficiency worldwide, especially in Third World countries.

Complementary Functions of World Markets

The poor countries of the South have no alternative than to become self-sufficient in food. The World markets can at best assume complementary functions. The countries would take indeterminable risks if they integrated themselves completely in the world markets, and thereby wanted to make themselves dependent upon global agro-markets. These are and will remain extremely unreliable factors that are conditioned by enormous fluctuations in prices and quantities, the powerful, and in many cases obscure, influences of multinational concerns, the manifold political interventions in the agricultural scene in most countries, and the dangers of social and ecological dumping.

But when we now look at the results of the WTO, we are disappointed. The development question and the balancing of hunger and surplus are finally no longer on the agenda. Programmes to increase food production in the poor countries were not the priority of the negotiations. The liberalization of agro-policies in the developing countries would have meant making the disadvantaging of their farmers the subject of international negotiations. That did not happen.

On the contrary, the concepts developed with an eye on the reform of agricultural policy of the North, which target the reduction of the support level, are to be transferred to the South without questions. To be sure, there are a whole number of exemptions for the poorest developing countries. But the WTO results have also set the trend there, namely the dismantlement of subsides. We cannot understand how such a thing can be demanded as a policy programme, especially for Africa. Support for African agriculture is largely absent, i.e. there is absolutely nothing to dismantle. That's why many international conferences repeatedly emphasize the need for these countries to achieve a greater degree of self-sufficiency in food by stronger support of their agriculture.

Agro-Dumping

Certainly, some changes have been made in the North's agro policy system which will also have positive impacts on world agricultural markets. However, also here we must express our disappointment. Agricultural dumping will continue. The only difference will be the new policy instrument of direct transfer of income instead of subsidized grain prices. The opening of markets in future will hardly go beyond the current preference conditions.

The entire set of W.T.O. agreements, however, bears the imprint of the two agricultural superpowers, the USA and the European Union, which make mutual concessions and coordinate their agricultural policies. But one hears nothing about the target of freeing the world agricultural market from unnecessary distortions and ensuring justice. The intention of the agro-superpowers was solely to defend their global market shares.

The development aid agencies cannot close their eyes to these problems. On the contrary, in future they must make very much greater efforts in suggesting better goals, programmes and instruments which are capable of forming a policy that can then be included in the agenda of the next rounds of negotiations. We may perhaps have slept a bit through the past WTO talks. Therefore it is even more important that we get very much more involved from now on.

6

Food Security: Availability and Access to Food

The world food situation has never been better. Enough food is being produced today that, if it were evenly distributed, no one should have to go hungry. World food production is increasing faster than population growth: per capita production increased by 5 per cent during the 1980s. Real food prices are at historic lows and have been declining for some time now. Yields of major cereals have more than doubled in the past three decades. These trends have contributed to complacency in some quarters regarding the world food situation.

Yet, more than 700 million people in the developing world do not have access to sufficient food to lead healthy and productive lives. More than 180 million children are underweight. Diseases of hunger and malnutrition are widespread. The desire to satisfy food needs has, in combination with increasing population densities and inadequate agricultural intensification, led to much degradation of environmentally fragile lands, such as forests and steep hillsides.

Over the next 20-30 years, farmers and policy makers in developing countries with be challenged to provide food at affordable prices for almost 100 million more people every year—the largest annual population increase in history. Moreover, they will have to increases food production from more productive use of the land and without further degradation of natural resources: area expansion is no longer a feasible option in most of the world.

What future food security will look like depends not on exogenous factors over which we have no control but on the decisions and actions taken by the major players: households, private—and public-sector agencies, governments, and the international community. If we continue to act as we have in the 1980s and early 1990s, more people will suffer from food insecurity, it will be because some or all of these players failed to act in an appropriate and timely manner.

Feeding the World: Availability and Access to Food

There is enough food in the world today to feed everyone, if it were evenly distributed. Availability of daily food energy per capita in the developing countries as a whole increased by 0.7 per cent per year during the 1980s.

Twenty-five developing countries, including about half of the African countries, were unable to assure sufficient food energy (2,200 calories per person per day) for their populations at the end of the 1980s even if available food energy were evenly distributed within each country. This is down from 45 countries at the end of the 1970s.

However, available food is neither evenly distributed nor fully consumed. Availability of enough food at global, regional, or national levels does not necessarily mean that everyone is well fed. For people to be food secure—that is, to have access at all times to the food required for a healthy and productive life—there must be both availability of food and access to food. Access to food by households (and individuals) is conditioned by poverty: the poor usually lack adequate means to secure access to food.

Over 1.1 billion people in developing countries were living in poverty in 1993, more than 500 million in conditions of extreme poverty. South Asia is the home of about 50 per cent of the developing world's poor—more than 500 million people. Another 15 per cent are found in East Asia, 19 per cent in Sub-Saharan Africa, and 10 per cent in Latin America and the Caribbean. The prevalence of poverty (the proportion of each region's population that is poor) is very high-about 50 per cent -in South Asia as well as in Sub-Saharan Africa.

Today, there are more than 700 million people who do not have access to sufficient food to meet their needs for a healthy and productive life; they often go hungry adults and children also suffer from diseases associated with hunger and poverty. For almost one fifth of the total population of developing countries to be chronically hungry tarnishes the image of a world that is now considered food-secure because it produces enough food.

Great progress has been made in meeting food needs during the last 30 years. For instance, the number of underfed people declined from an estimated 976 million in 1974-76 to 786 million in late 1980s. But the problem is far from solved. Keeping up with increasing needs and demands due to population growth, income increases, and dietary changes is itself a formidable challenge.

Hunger and food insecurity have a significant effect on health and nutrition of both adults and children. They can lead to growth failure in children. About 184 million preschool children in developing countries were underweight in 1994. About 55 per cent of these underweight children were found in South Asia and another 16 per cent in Sub-Saharan Africa. The proportion of children that are underweight is higher in South Asia (almost 60 per cent), but it is also significant in Sub-Saharan Africa (30 per cent) and Southeast Asia (31 per cent). It is worrisome that the number of underweight children in Sub-Saharan Africa during the 1980s from [illegible] million to 28 million is particularly striking.

In addition to energy deficiencies, micro nutrient deficiencies are also widespread in the developing world. About 14 million preschool children (under the age of five years) have eye damage as a result of vitamin A deficiency.

Ten million of these children are found in Southeast Asia. Between 250,000 and 500,000 preschool children go blind each year due to vitamin A deficiency, two-thirds of these children die within months of going blind. Many more children are mildly affected. Recent research has shown that even mild deficiencies can increase mortality significantly. Vitamin A deficiencies are closely linked to diet, which can be influenced by agricultural research and policy.

Iron deficiency affects about 1 billion people in the world, particularly children and women of reproductive age. Iron deficiency leads to anemia, which if not checked can diminish learning capacity and increase morbidity and morality. In the developing countries, about 370 million women between 15 and 49 years of age—42 per cent of this population group—were anemic in the 1980s. Almost one-half were in South Asia. And there are tentative indications from South Asia and Sub-Saharan Africa that the prevalence of anemia is rising in non pregnant adult women of reproductive ages.

In Sub-Saharan Africa, this trend is undoubtedly associated with deterioration in general standards of living, including increased poverty and food insecurity. Anemia partly arises from diets insufficient in iron, which again could be addressed through agricultural research and policy. For example, a possible reason why iron deficiency and anemia are going up in South Asia may lie in the decrease in production of iron rich pulses during that same period, which in part reflects the larger research input into competing crops such as wheat in South Asia. This emphasizes the importance of considering the effects on died and thus on health and nutrition in setting research priorities for yield-increasing research.

South Asia is the home of about half of the developing world's hungry and food-insecure people, but this population group is growing rapidly in Sub-Saharan Africa. Much of the poverty and food insecurity is in rural areas, mainly in low-potential areas such as arid zones, but urban poverty is also growing rapidly.

Four Key Factors will Influence Future Food Production and Consumption

Global and regional food production consumption during the next 10-20 years will be influenced by a large number of factors. Changes in the following four sets of Actors are likely to particularly important:

1. Economic growth and economic policies.
2. Population growth and urbanization.
3. Rural infrastructure, agricultural production technology, and access to modern inputs, and
4. Natural resource management and environmental considerations.

The expected impact of each of these factors on future food production and consumption is considerable.

Economic Growth and Economic Policies

Economic growth must resume in the developing world, especially in Sub-Saharan Africa. To support such growth, it is critical to

- complete structural adjustment and economic reforms;
- remove external barriers to growth such as trade distortions and subsidies in developed countries;
- liberalize trade and remove market distortions;
- enhance access by the poor to land, capital, and technology;
- expand investment in rural infrastructure, health, education, and agricultural research and technology;
- facilitate sustainability in agricultural production and
- reverse the decline in international assistance to agriculture.

Growth in real per capita income during the 1980s was disappointing for developing countries as a whole. However, the low average rate of growth covers large variations among regions. The high rates of economic growth in Asia are expected to continue through the 1990s, while incomes in Sub-Saharan Africa are expected to keep pace with population growth.

Future economic growth depends on internal policies as well as on the international policies as well as on the international environment. The extent to which current structural adjustment and economic reforms in Latin America, Sub-Saharan Africa, the Commonwealth of Independent States (CIS), Eastern Europe, and selected countries in Asia and the Middle East are carried to successful completion at an appropriate speed and sequence is of paramount importance for future economic growth in those countries.

Closely related to this issue is the question of the most appropriate role of the state in a market-oriented economy with inappropriate institutions, poor infrastructure, and insufficient experience by the private sector in dealing effectively in a competitive market environment. Overreaction to past failures such as excessive and inappropriate state intervention may cause governments to take on a passive role where intervention is needed to assure that the markets function effectively and to deal with outside influences on the economy.

Future economic growth will also depend on the international trade environment, including trade distortions by developed countries, and access to external aid. Import restrictions for agricultural and nonagricultural products in Japan, the European Union, and the United States, along with domestic agricultural subsidies and implicit and explicit export subsidies for agricultural products, are of particular concern.

Population Growth and Urbanization

If progress in economic growth is not to be undermined by rapid population growth and excessive urbanization, effective population and migration policies are necessary to complement growth-oriented policies. Such policies must focus on

- universal access to family planning information and technology; and
- incentives to reduce rural-urban migration, such as provision of employment in rural areas and stimulation of agricultural and nonagricultural growth in rural areas.

Although the annual growth rate is falling for the world as a whole, the population increase during the next 20-30 years, of slightly less than 100 million people a year, will be the largest ever. Approximately 97 per cent of this increase is projected to occur in the Third World, with Africa alone accounting for 34 per cent of the growth. Thus although reductions in annual population growth rates have begun to occur in Asia and Latin America, they are insufficient to counter the absolute increases. Population growth rates of these magnitudes will greatly increase the need for food and other basic necessities.

Rural Infrastructure, Agricultural Production Technology, and Access to Modern Inputs

Continued progress in all three of these areas is critical to future food security.

- Resources must be committed to infrastructure construction and maintenance. Labor-intensive public works programmes are a viable mechanism for building roads, reforesting areas, and engaging in soil conservation projects, while creating employment and income in rural areas.
- International and national agricultural research must continue to develop yield-enhancing production technology, especially in maize, millet, and other crops, as well as build tolerance or resistance in crops to pests and adverse climatic conditions.

> Farmer access to modern inputs must be facilitated through provision of credit and technical assistance. Inputs must be made available to all farmers on time and in required amounts.

The importance of investments in rural infrastructure within the context of rapid urbanization has already been established. Even without rapid urban growth, however, such investments are needed in many developing countries, particularly the poorest ones, to facilitate agricultural and rural development. Improved rural infrastructure enhances access to export markets, modern production inputs, and consumer goods. It reduces marketing costs, promotes exchange between intracountry markets, reduces spatial and temporal price distortions, and, in general, increases efficiency in production and marketing.

However, while essential, effective rural infrastructure alone is not enough to assure agricultural and rural development and rapid increases in food production in developing countries. Yield enhancing production technology is of critical importance. Although opportunities for expansion of agricultural production into lands not currently under cultivation still exist in some countries, such opportunities are so limited that they would probably not be able to counter losses of current agricultural lands to alternative uses on a global level. Furthermore, attempts to expand agricultural production into new lands would, in most cases, require large investments in technology, tools and materials and would increase the risk of land degradation and deforestation. Thus, future increases in food production must come primarily from higher yields per unit of land rather than from land expansion.

Agricultural research has successfully developed yield-enhancing technology for the majority of crops grown in temperate zones and for several crops grown in tropical zones. The dramatic impact of agricultural research and modern technology on wheat and rice yields in Asia and Latin America since the mid-1980s is well known. Less dramatic but significant yield gains have been obtained from research and technological change in other crops, particularly maize.

Natural Resource Management and Environmental Considerations

Research, technology development, incentives, and regulations are needed to prevent environmental degradation. These measures include appropriate water management policies, reduction of subsidies that encourage wasteful use of inputs, better definition of ownership and user rights to resources including land, education of farmers to encourage appropriate use of technology and resource conservation, and the provision of alternatives to resource-degrading inputs and techniques. Since poverty is a major source of degradation, poverty eradication is justified also on environmental grounds.

The recent surge in public and private concerns about negative environmental effects of economic growth and development may, if sustained, have important implications for agricultural development and future food production and consumption. Of particular concern of the need to avoid degradation of natural resources such as land and water, as well as deforestation, water contamination, and health risks associated with the use of chemicals. Since most of the current and potential resource degradation and environmental contamination result from situations in which those who cause and possibly benefit from degradation do not pay the costs, neither the market nor the individual producers and consumers are likely to incorporate preventive measures into their behaviour. Only when sufficient damage has been done to influence significantly current or future production costs will market and producer behaviour change. The state is more likely to undertake preventive measures either through publicly funded research and technology development or through incentive policies and regulations. Extensive water logging, salination, and associated land degradation and productivity losses resulting from inappropriate water management are of particular concern in large parts of Asia.

No Time for Complacency

Population growth will outstrip growth in food production in Sub-Saharan Africa for a long time to come unless more is done to accelerate agricultural growth. Between now and 2000, the population will grow at more than 3 per cent a year, while food production is likely to grow at 2 per cent or less a year. By the year 2000, the production shortfall is estimated to increase to about 50 million tons of grain equivalent, up from the current level of about 14 million tons. The region will not have the necessary foreign exchange to import such large amounts of food. And African governments will not be able to count on enough food aid to make up the difference. If current trends continue, by the year 2020, Africa will have a food shortage of 250 million tons, which is more than 20 times the current food gap.

Poverty is expected to increase rapidly in the coming years. Sub-Saharan Africa's share of the world's poor is expected to increase from the current 19 per cent to about 28 per cent in 2000. Furthermore, the number of underweight children in expected to increase in the 1990's in Sub-Saharan Africa.

Asian demand for cereals is estimated to grow at an annual rate of 2.1 per cent between now and the year 2000, where as food production is expected to grow at 1.9 per cent per year. Much of the production shortfall is likely to be dealt with through expanded imports and perhaps through expanded regional production in response to price increases.

In Latin America, by contrast, growth in food production is anticipated to exceed food demand growth: food production is estimated to grow by 3 per cent annually between 1990 and 2000, while food demand is estimated to grow by 2.5 per cent per year.

Large areas of land are rapidly being degraded and deforested. And the principal reasons for environmental degradation–poverty, high population growth, and limited access to appropriate agricultural technology–are not being dealt with effectively.

About 700 million people are food insecure for them the food crisis has arrived. For the 10-12 million preschool children who died in 1994 from hunger and diseases related to malnutrition, the food crisis came and went. One-third of the preschool children of the Third World are unable to grow to their full potential and face increased risk of death and disease.

Complacency is not in order. Clearly, Malthus underestimated the power of science to expand food production. The mass starvation that was predicted for Asia in the 1970s and 1980s did not occur because science was effectively put to work to expand crop yields. However, past yield increases came about people with foresight made appropriate decisions. The failure to expand investments in agricultural research and technology development during the 1980s and 1990s indicates that such foresight no longer prevails. Given the long lag time between investment in agricultural research and the resulting production increases, failure to invest today will show up in production shortfalls 10 to 20 years from now. The problems associated with environmental degradation will present themselves sooner. We must not wait until a global food crisis is upon us or until the last tree has fallen to make these investments.

References

1. FAO, *FAO Production Yearbook.*
2. FAO, *"The State of Food and Agriculture 1992".*
3. FAO, *"Agriculture Towards 2010".*
4. FAO, *"The State of Food and Agriculture 1994".*
5. FAO, *Food Outlook (December 1994).*
6. World Bank, *World Development Report 1995.*
7. World Bank, *Global Economic Prospects and the Developing Countries.*
8. World Food Programme, *Food Aid in Review (Rome: WFP 1992).*
9. World Bank, *Global Economic Prospects and the Developing Countries 1992* (Washington, D.C.: World Bank).

7

Genetic Diversity and Food Security

Maintaining a diversity of crops and varieties is a key to survival for millions of farmers living on impoverished land. For thousands of years, farmers have used the genetic variation in wild and cultivated plants to develop their crops and raise new breeds of live stock. Genetic diversity gives species the ability to adapt to changing environments, including new pests and diseases and new climatic conditions. Plant genetic resources—that component of genetic diversity of actual or potential use to humanity—provide the raw material for breeding new varieties of crops. These, in turn, provide a basis for more productive and resilient production systems that are better able to cope with such stresses as drought or overgrazing and can reduce the potential for soil erosion. The use of genetic diversity—on-farm, through field experimentation or in sophisticated gene transfer procedures—remains arguably the best route so securing our food and that of our children.

Although science has made enormous strides in improving the world" ability to feed itself over the past three decades, we cannot afford to rest idle. Nearly 800 million people in the developing world do not have enough to eat. In these regions, the rural poor represent about 73 per cent of the people living in poverty. They often live in marginal or unsuitable farming areas, such as zones with saline soils, and conditions, or degraded or hilly areas. Often isolated from others farms and far from urban areas, many poor farmers have barely benefited from agricultural developments elsewhere. In many cases they do not have access to commercially bred high yielding crop varieties. Diversity flourishes and remains important under such conditions.

Selections and Breeding

Poor farmers are well aware of the relationship between the stability and sustainability of crops and crop varieties on their lands. Their management and use of a diverse range of plants has often helped them to survive under the most difficult conditions. By growing a range of different crops, farmers have a better chance of meeting their needs. These might be crops that mature at different times or that can be easily stored to help to ensure a stable food supply throughout the year. They may also help farmers provide a nutritionally balance diet for their families, exploit different environment niches that exist on their land, or diversify their income sources.

Importantly, the genetic diversity contained in different varieties provides farmers with options to develop, through selection and breeding, new and more productive crops that are resistant to pests and diseases. The result may be a vast range of local varieties of crops grown by farmers in any one area.

Not respecting diversity can incur high costs: in 18th century Ireland, where potatoes were the only significant source of food for about one third of the population, farmers came to rely almost entirely on one very fertile and productive variety, which proved susceptible to the devastating potato blight fungus. The resulting famine caused the death or emigration of more than 20 per cent of the population.

The value of diversity goes well beyond its ability to support stable production systems in marginal environments. As the world's human population rises, environmental problems (desertification, deforestation, erosion etc.) are intensifying, Climate change, particularly global warming, could bring about drastic changes in the location of the world's agro-ecological zones. Farmers will require new crop varieties capable of producing under diverse conditions, without adding ever-increasing amounts of fertilizers and other agro-chemicals. Because of the limited scope for growth in the world's cultivated areas, each new generation of varieties will have to be more productive than its predecessors.

Much has been written about the use of genetic engineering in plant breeding. Modern molecular techniques can be used to transfer genes from one living organism to another or to change the genetic material within to produce more desirable traits. Genetic Engineering has enormous potential to help solve problems that have proved intractable using conventional breeding approaches, such as developing crop varieties with in-built resistance to key pests and diseases and tolerance to stresses such as drought. However, the possible impact of these techniques, particularly on human health and the environment, is giving rise to fierce worlds wide debate.

Take the case of banana and its close relative plantain, two of the developing world's most important crops. Their improvement is hindered by the sterility of most cultivars, a problem that can be addressed through genetic engineering. It is now possible to transfer gene constructs, such as those associated with disease resistance, directly into varieties with other desirable characteristics, drastically reducing the need for pesticides.

Today, research on genetic engineering is focussed on the development of commercial varieties of the world's major crops of interest to industrialized farmers. Many of the staple crops of importance to poor farmers in developing countries, such as cassava, bananas, beans and yams, have received relatively little attention. This situation is likely to continue as plant breeding is increasingly privatized and biotechnology becomes the fast-growing province of private industry. Meanwhile, the high costs of the new technologies are quickly exceeding the capacity of many, if not most, public research institutions—both in developing and developed countries—to support them. Thus, for the time being, increasing agriculture's role in the development of the world's poor is likely to continue to depend on the identification, maintenance and use of genetic diversity.

8

Population Growth and Grain Production

The relationship between the growth in world population and the grain harvest has shifted over the last half-century, neatly dividing this period into two distinct eras. From 1950 to 1984, growth and the grain harvest easily exceeded that of population, raising the harvest per person from 247 kilograms to 342, a gain of 38 per cent. During the 14 years since then, growth in the grain harvest has fallen behind that of population, dropping output per person from its historic high in 1984 to an estimated 317 kilograms in 1998—a decline of 7 per cent, or 0.5 per cent a year.

These global trends conceal widely divergent developments among countries, contrasts that can be seen for the world's two most populous nations: India and China. In both, grain production per person was close to 200 kilograms as recently as 1978. Since then, the figure in India has edged up slightly but still falls short of 200 kilograms, while in china production has surged since the economic reforms in 1978, with per-person output now at nearly 300 kilograms. The combination of a dramatic surge in grain production and an equally dramatic reduction in population growth has given China a large margin of safety, effectively eliminating most of its hunger and malnutrition. Meanwhile, although India has also achieved impressive gains in its harvest, these have been largely cancelled by population growth, leaving its 976 million people living close to the margin.

What has happened in China and India is the story of developing countries in general. The overwhelming majority have achieved substantial, if not dramatic, gains in their grain harvests over the last half-century. Some, such as Thailand, have combined this with a much slower growth of population, which means that agricultural gains translate into rising grain production per person. In Pakistan, by contrast, grain production per person climbed steadily for a while, but it peaked in 1981 at 186 kilograms. Since then it has been declining nearly 1 per cent a year. In effect, Pakistan's farmers are losing the battle with population growth.

The slower growth in the world grain harvest since 1984 is due to the lack of new land and to slower growth in irrigation and fertilizer use. Irrigated area per person, after expanding by 4 per cent since then as growth in the irrigated area has fallen behind that of population.

The increase in world fertilizer use has slowed dramatically since 1990, as diminishing returns to the application of additional fertilizer has stabilized use in the United States, Western Europe, and Japan and slowed annual growth in world fertilizer use from 6 per cent between 1950 and 1990 to scarcely 2 per cent in recent years.

Although Malthus was primarily concerned with the additional demand for grain generated by population growth, rising affluence is also playing a role. In a low income country such as India, grain consumption per person is less than 200 kilograms per year and diets are typically dominated by a single starchy staple-rice, for instance. With scarcely a pound of grain available a day per person, nearly all must be consumed directly, leaving little for conversion into animal protein. For the average American, on the other hand, the great bulk of the 800-kilogam daily grain consumption is taken in indirectly in the form of beef, pork, poultry, eggs, milk, cheese, ice cream, and yogurt. At the intermediate level, in a country like Italy, people consume 400 kilograms of grain a day. Future food price stability thus depends on expanding production fast enough to keep up with both population growth and rising affluence.

One question often asked is, How many people can the Earth support? This must be answered with another question, At what level of consumption? If the world grain harvest of 1.87 billion tons were expanded to 2 billion tons in the years ahead, it would support 10 billion Indians or 2.5 billion Americans. To answer the question of how many people the Earth can support, we first have to know the level of consumption we expect to live at.

Now that the frontiers of agricultural settlement have disappeared, future growth in grain production must come almost entirely from raising land productivity. Unfortunately, this is becoming more difficult. After rising at 2.1 per cent a year from 1950 to 1990, the annual increase in rainland productivity dropped to scarcely 1 per cent from 1990 to 1997. The challenge for the world's farmers is to reverse this decline at a time when cropland area per person is shrinking, the amount of irrigation water per person is dropping, and the crop yield response to additional fertilizer use is falling.

9

Population Growth and Cropland

Since mid-century, global population has grown much faster than the cropland area. The trend is likely to continue in the next century, dropping cropland per person to historically low levels. The ever smaller per capita cropland base will make food self-sufficiency impossible for many countries, and will test the capacity of international markets to meet a growing demand for imported food.

For millennia, farmers satisfied rising food demand by bringing new land under the plow. But by mid-century cropland expansion could no longer meet the food needs of an increasingly populous and prosperous world. The 10,000 year era of steady expansion was over, a new era began that stressed raising land productivity. As this high-yielding era shows signs of faltering, concern over the shrinking supply of cropland per person looms ever larger.

Since mid-century, grain area-which serves as a proxy for cropland in general-has increased by some 19 per cent, but global population has grown 132 per cent, seven times faster. Largely as a result, grain area per person has fallen by half since 1950, from 0.24 to 0.12 hectares. Assuming that grain area remains constant, grain area per person will fall to 0.07 hectares by 2050. In crowded industrial countries such as Japan, Taiwan, and South Korea, grain area per capita today is smaller than the area of a tennis court.

As grain area per person falls, more and more nations risk losing the capacity to feed themselves. Having already seen per capita grain area shrink by 40-50 per cent between 1960 and 1998, Pakistan, Nigeria, Ethiopia, and Iran can expect a further 60-70 per cent loss by 2050-a conservative projection that assumes no further losses of agricultural land. The result will be four countries with a combined population of more than 1 billion whose grain area per person will be only 300-600 square metres, less than a quarter of the area in 1950.

The historical record suggests that such a small area per person will send a substantial share of a country's people to world markets from their food. Consider the experience of six countries in East Asia whose per capita grain area currently ranges from 200 to 600 square metres per person. Sri Lanka relies on imports for more than a third of its grain, while Japan, Taiwan, South Korea, and Malaysia buy more than 70 per cent of their grain from abroad. North Korea is the only one of the six that does not import heavily (it gets less than 20 per cent of its grain requirements from abroad), but its population is poorly fed-indeed, on the verge of starvation.

The concern is that population growth will push many nations—not just the four fastest-growing ones—below the 600-square metre-threshold in coming decades. In Asia alone, where grain area per person stands at 800 square metres, 16 countries are poised to cross this threshold by 2050, and many of them much sooner. As this process unfolds, the number of people who will turn to foreign markets for their food will likely jump sharply. These countries will find an increasingly tight international grain market, with nations from the Middle East, North Africa, and other regions already buying a third or more of their grain overseas.

In addition to per capita losses, population growth can lead to degradation of cropland, reducing its productivity or even eliminating it from production. As a country's population density increases and good farmland becomes scarce, poor farmers are forced onto ecologically vulnerable land such as hillsides and tropical forest. In the Philippines, for example, hillside agriculture accounted for only 10 per cent of all agricultural land in 1960, but 30 per cent in 1987. Because it is highly erodible, hillside land is easily damaged; worldwide, some 160 million hectares of hillside farmland—11 per cent of cropland-were characterized in 1989 as "severely eroded." Similarly, population pressure can force peasants to overfarm the poor soils of tropical forests. After being cleared and farmed for a few years, these soils typically require fallow periods of 20-25 years, but population pressures keep poor farmers on the same land for far longer than the soil can support, cutting fallow periods to just a few years in some areas of tropical Africa and Asia.

Finally, population pressures on a fixed base of land can result in rural landlessness. In Bangladesh, for example, landlessness among rural households rose from 35 per cent in 1960 to 53 per cent in the early 1990s. Interestingly, Bangladesh is regarded as a success in slowing population expansion, as its growth rate declined from 2.8 per cent in the late 1970s to 1.5 per cent in the early 1990s. But its success came too late to prevent the increase in rural landlessness, highlighting the need to work sooner, rather than later, for population stabilization.

10

Population Growth and Oceanic Fish Catch

From 1950 until 1988, the oceanic fish catch soared from 19 million to 88 million tons, expanding much faster than population. The per capita catch increased from less than 8 kilograms in 1950 to the historical peak of just over 17 kilograms in 1988, more than doubling since 1988, however, growth in the catch has slowed, falling behind that of population. Between 1988 and 1996, the catch per person declined to less than 16 kilograms, a drop of some 9 per cent.

This five fold growth in the human appetite for sea food since 1950 has pushed the catch of most oceanic fisheries to their sustainable limits or beyond. Marine biologists believe that the oceans cannot sustain an annual catch of much more than 93 million tons, the current take.

As we near the end of the twentieth century, overfishing has become the rule, not the exception. Of the 15 major oceanic fisheries. 11 are in decline. The catch of Atlantic cod-long a dietary mainstay for West Europeans—has fallen by some 70 per cent since peaking in 1968. Since 1970, Bluefin Tuna stocks in the West Atlantic have dropped 80 per cent.

The next half-century is likely to be marked by the disappearance of some species from markets, a decline in the quality of seafood caught, higher prices, and more conflicts among countries over access to fisheries. Over the last two decades, a growing share of the catch has consisted of inferior species, some of which were not even considered edible in times past.

The growing scarcity of the species at the top of the food chain is reflected in rising prices. Poor people who once ate fish because they could not afford meat now find that meat is often less expensive than seafood. Although most price rises are moderate, some are extreme-going far beyond anything we could have earlier imagined. The decline of the Bluefin Tuna population in the Atlantic, for instance, has occasionally pushed prices for a 300-Kilogram Tuna above $80,000 at top-of-the-line Sushi restaurants in Japan compete for the few of these giant fish that are available.

This growing competition for limited resources has led to ongoing conflicts among countries. The United Nations recorded more than 100 such disputes in 1997. These are evident in the cod wars between Norwegian and Icelandic ships, between Canada and Spain over turbot off Canada's eastern coast, between China and the Marshall Islands in Micronesia, between Argentina and Taiwan over Falkland island fisheries, and between Indonesia and the Philippines in the Celebes. There are "Tuna wars in the northeast Atlantic, Crab wars in the North Pacific, Squid wars in the southwest Atlantic, Salmon wars in the North Pacific, and Pollock wars in the Sea of Okhotsk." Although these disputes make it into the world news only rarely, they are now an almost daily occurrence. Indeed, historians may record more fishery conflicts during one year in the 1990s than during the entire nineteenth century.

One of the consequences of modern fishing technologies, whether it is the use of drift nets or bottom-scouring fish-catch of unwanted species. This oceanic equivalent of clearcutting is damaging fisheries on an unprecedented scale.

With the oceans now pushed to their limits, future growth in the demand for seafood can be satisfied only by fish farming. As a result, aquacultural output has increased from 7 million tons in 1984 to an estimated 26 million tons in 1977. Most of this growth in catch is based on just a few species, such as Carp, which constitute most of the aquacultural harvest in China, and Catfish, which dominates fish farming in the United States. As the world turns to fish farming to satisfy its needs, fish begin to compete with livestock and poultry for foodstuffs such as grain, soyabean meal, and fishmeal.

Given that the oceanic fish catch is apparently now at or beyond its sustainable limit, it is a relatively simple matter to determine the future oceanic catch per person. With each year, this will decline by roughly the amount of population growth, dropping to 9.9 kilograms per person in 2050, a decline to little more than half the 1988 peak of 17.2 kilograms. Those of us born before 1950 have enjoyed a doubling of the seafood catch per person, while those born in recent years are likely to witness a decline of nearly one half during their lifetimes.

11

The Uruguay Round and Agricultural Reform

The Uruguay Round of Multilateral trade negotiations (completed in 1994) continued the process of reducing trade barriers achieved in seven previous rounds of negotiations. Among the Uruguay Round's most significant accomplishments were the adoption of new rules governing agricultural trade policy, the establishment of disciplines on the use of Sanitary and Phytosanitary (SPS) measures, and agreement on a new process for settling trade disputes. The Uruguay Round also created the World Trade Organization (WTO) to replace the General Agreement on Tariffs and Trade (GATT) as an institutional framework for overseeing trade negotiations and adjudicating trade disputes. Agricultural trade concerns that have come to the fore since the Uruguay Round, including the use of genetically engineered products in agricultural trade, state trading, and a large number of potential new members, illustrate the wide range of issues any new round may face.

During the past years since initial implementation of the Uruguay Round agreements, the record with respect to agriculture is mixed: The Uruguay Round's overall impact on agricultural trade can be considered positive in moving toward several key goals, including reducing agricultural export subsidies, establishing new rules for agricultural import policy, and agreeing on disciplines for Sanitary and Phytosanitary trade measures. The Uruguay Round Agreement on Agriculture (URAA) may also have contributed to a shift in domestic support of agriculture away from those practices with the largest potential to affect production and, therefore, to affect trade flows. However, significant reductions in most agricultural tariffs will have to await a future round of negotiations.

Tariffs, Incentives, and Subsidies

Prior to Uruguay Round, trade in many agricultural products was unaffected by the tariff cuts that were made for industrial products in previous rounds. In the Uruguay Round, participating countries agreed to convert all nontariff agricultural trade barriers to tariffs (a process called "tariffication") and to reduce them. However, agricultural tariffs remain very high for some products in some countries, limiting the trade benefits to be derived from the new rules. To ensure that historical trade levels were maintained and to create some new trade opportunities where trade had been largely precluded by policies, countries instituted tariff-rate quotas. A tariff-rate quota applies a lower tariff to imports below a certain quantitative limit (quota) and permits a higher tariff on imported goods after the quota has been reached.

The Agreement on Agriculture required countries to reduce outlays on domestic policies that provide direct economic incentives to producers to increase resource use or production. All WTO member countries are meeting their commitments to reduce these outlays, and most countries reduced this type of support by more than the required amount. However, support from those domestic policies considered to have the least effect on production, such as domestic food aid, has increased from 1986-88 levels.

In the Agreement on Agriculture, 25 countries that employed export subsidies agreed to reduce the volume and value of their subsidized exports over a specified implementation period. To date, most of these countries have met their commitments, although some have found ways to circumvent them. The European Union (EU) is by far the largest user of export subsidies, accounting for 84 per cent of subsidy outlays of the 25 countries in 1995 and 1996. Despite substantial progress in reducing export subsidies, rising world grain supplies and falling world grain prices will make it difficult for some countries to meet future commitments unless they adopt policy changes.

The Uruguay Round's SPS agreement imposed disciplines on the use of measures to protect human, animal, and plant life and health from foreign pests, diseases, and contaminants. The agreement can be credited with increasing the transparency of countries SPS regulations and providing improved means for settling SPS-related trade disputes, including some important cases involving agricultural products. The agreement has also spurred regulatory reforms in some countries. The SPS agreement and the Agreement on Technical Barriers to Trade could provide a framework for disputes over genetically modified organisms (GMOs) brought to the WTO for arbitration.

Current Issues

Changes made to the multilateral dispute resolution process in the Uruguay Round may be as important to agricultural trade as the improvement in the substantive rules governing trade in agricultural goods. Initial evidence indicates that the WTO dispute settlement system is a significant improvement over its GATT predecessor. For example, a single country can no longer block the formation of a dispute resolution panel or veto an adverse ruling by blocking the adoption of a panel report. These improvements have led to a number of important agricultural trade cases being adjudicated before the WTO. The outstanding question for the WTO is whether members whose practices have been successfully challenged under the new dispute settlement procedures will live up to their obligations.

Other agriculture-related issues, including a bid for membership by a large and diverse group of potential new

WTO members, the challenge of dealing with state trading enterprises (STEs) within WTO disciplines, and issues particular to developing countries, will shape the agenda for future agricultural trade liberalization discussions. Thirty countries are currently seeking membership in the 134-member WTO. Countries seeking WTO membership accede under conditions negotiated with WTO membership through the privileged trade status with WTO member but may incur adjustment costs in reforming their trade policies and reducing tariffs to meet WTO requirements. Current WTO members gain greater access to the markets of acceding countries.

State trading enterprises, governmental and non-governmental entities that have been granted special rights or privileges through which they can influence trade, continue to be important to the trade of agricultural commodities because many countries consider them to be an appropriate means to meet domestic agricultural policy objectives. Continuing concerns about the trade practices of state trading enterprises in some WTO member countries and the potential accession of China and other countries where STEs are prominent will keep STEs on the WTO agenda.

Developing countries received special treatment in the Uruguay Round, including less stringent disciplines in reforming their trade policies than those apply to developed countries. In the next round of multilateral agricultural trade negotiations, developing countries will continue to have their own interests in the areas of special and differential treatment, export restraints, price stability, food security, food aid, and stock policies. As developing countries identify their positions, coalitions of countries with common trade interests may emerge.

12

Developing Countries and the WTO Agricultural Negotiations

Developing countries as a group have much to gain from continued progress toward a transparent, rule-based trading system in agriculture. The researches say the negotiations should eliminate export subsidies, impose stricter disciplines on export taxes, cut tariffs, and ensure that food aid continues to be available to poor countries in grant form and delivered so as not to displace domestic production in the countries receiving it. Badly managed food aid, or cheap food imports due to export subsidies, may just reinforce the bias of economic policies against the rural sector. With its negative impact on poor agricultural producers, "they say. International research organizations (such as IFPRI, among other institutions) may provide support to developing countries through programmes of collaborative research, technical assistance, and capacity strengthening.

Starting with the first round of trade negotiations under the General Agreement on Tariffs and Trade (GATT) after World War II, there has been a relatively steady trend of increasing multilateral trade liberalization. The successive rounds of negotiations recognized the greater needs of developing countries, especially since the Tokyo Round. Yet the participation of developing countries was limited. Since many developing countries were not members of GATT, the major forum for airing their views was provided by the United Nations Conference on Trade and Development. The views of developing countries had some impact on the Lome agreements and on aid flows, but had limited influence on negotiations concerning trading rules, which were discussed within the framework of the GATT, where OECD (Organization for Economic Cooperation and Development) countries set the agenda.

In the Uruguay Round, which began in 1986 and concluded in 1993, developing countries played a larger role in the negotiations compared to previous rounds. In particular, agricultural net exporters organized the Cairns Group (which in addition to Australia, New Zealand, and Canada, included several large developing countries such as Argentina, Brazil, Indonesia, and the Philippines) to pursue their interests. Furthermore, during and after the conclusion of the Uruguay Round, the formal accession of developing countries to the GATT and now the World Trade Organization (WTO) has continued apace. Of the 134 members of the WTO in February 1999, some 70 per cent were developing countries. The United Nations classified 48 countries as least-developed (LLDCs). Within that group, 29 are members of the WTO, six are in the process of accession, and three are observers. Also, 18 countries have been identified as net-food-importing developing countries (NFIDCs).

Some Definitions

The LLDCs are identified by the United Nations General Assembly based on several criteria—income per capita, augmented physical quality of life index, and an index of economic diversification. As a group, they have a population of about 590 million people, with an income per capita about 4 per cent that of the world average (1996). Agricultural production per capita in LLDCs has been declining since the 1970s although the same indicator for all developing countries (mainly under the influence of China) has gone up by nearly 40 per cent in the same period. LLDCs represent a small fraction of world trade (less than 1 per cent for total and about 2 per cent for agricultural trade). They had a positive, although declining net agricultural trade balance until the mid 1980s, when it turned negative. Almost 20 per cent of their total imports are food items.

The 18 net-food-importing developing countries have been selected through a process within the WTO. They have a population of some 380 million people and an income per capita nearly five time that of the LLDC average, but still much lower than the world average. NFIDCs are a diverse group: four are upper-middle income countries; eight are lower-middle income; and six are lower income. Four of them had net food exports on average during 1995-97, but because they imported cereals they are included in the group. NFIDCs' per capita food production as share of both world and developing country averages has risen, although from very low levels.

Although the categories of "developed" and "developing" countries have important legal consequences under WTO rules, there are no formal definitions of either category. The process works through self-identification and negotiation with other member countries of the WTO.

Completing the Unfinished Agenda

In general, developing countries operate under what has been called "special and differential treatment". They face lower disciplines and enjoy longer time frames for implementing reforms. In the case of LLDCs, they are totally exempted from WTO commitments, and it has been agreed that developing and least-developed countries should receive special consideration for market access and technical and financial support. Also, during the Uruguay Round, concerns that liberalization of agricultural policies and trade could adversely affect the food imports of LLDCs and NFIDCs led participants to include several measures dealing with food security issues in the "green box" of permitted domestic support—for instance, the formation of public stockholding and the provision of foodstuffs at subsidized prices. There was a ministerial decision in Marrakesh in April 1994 to deal with possible negative effects of agricultural trade reforms on the food security of LLDCs and NFIDCs. The decision was reemphasized at the 1996 ministerial meeting of the WTO in Singapore.

Export and Domestic Subsidies: While many developing countries have significantly reduced distorting domestic agricultural policies, the possible benefits that these countries and the world can enjoy are thwarted by the subsidies of developed countries. The Uruguay Round was a first step in imposing discipline on the unfair competition arising from subsidized agricultural exports, which hurts poor agricultural producers in developing countries irrespective of their net agricultural trade position. In the next negotiations, that first step should be completed with the elimination of export subsidies. Net-food-importing developing countries should also be interested in stricter disciplines on export taxes and controls that exacerbate price fluctuations in world markets.

Under the Uruguay Round agreement, there is still a lot of scope for the developed countries to use domestic subsidies, in addition to the use of export subsidies; to help their farmers. The developing countries should seek further disciplines in this regard, including, among other things, the elimination of exemptions under the “blue box” (which allows farmers to receive some forms of direct payments that are considered to be trade distorting). Least-developed and developing countries, however, will still be allowed “special and differential treatment” on these issues.

Market Access: If the developing countries are to succeed in diversifying their agricultural sectors, they need expanded access to markets in developed countries. This includes increasing the volume of imports allowed under the current regime of tariff-rate quotas (TRQs), which replaced the previous system of rigid quotas with a combination of a quantitative quota and a high tariff for the eventual out-of-quota imports); making the administration of the TRQs more transparent and equitable; seeking further reductions in tariffs, particularly those still high in some key products; and completing the process of tariffication in the cases where exemptions were granted. Also, eliminating, or at least reducing, tariff escalation in nonagricultural products is important for developing countries: this practice undermines the possibilities of expanding production and exports of processed goods that use agricultural inputs, exploiting "forward linkages" in the value-added chain.

What the Most Vulnerable Need

The special situation and concerns of least-developed countries and net-food-importing countries were recognized in a ministerial decision agreed upon at the completion of the Uruguay Round in 1993. These concerns include the preservation of adequate levels of food aid, the provision of technical assistance and financial support to develop the agricultural sector in those countries, and the continuation and expansion of financial facilities to help with structural adjustment and short-term difficulties in financing food imports. It is important to make food aid available in grant form, to target it to poor countries and social groups, and to deliver it in ways that do not displace domestic production in the countries receiving it. Badly managed food aid, or cheap food imports due to export subsidies, may just reinforce the bias of economic policies against the rural sector, with its negative impact on poor agricultural producers.

Volatility in agricultural prices must be monitored carefully. While expansion of world agricultural trade should limit overall fluctuations by spreading supply and demand stocks over larger areas, the decline in world public stocks as a percentage of consumption works in the opposite direction. Improving early warning of potential food shortages, lowering costs for food transportation and storage, and providing better targeted food aid programmes and financial facilities for emergencies are also issues that need to be addressed by countries participating in the coming round of negotiations.

The impact of changes in trade and agricultural policy on poorer consumers and producers in developing countries is a matter of debate. Some have argued that trade liberalization may hurt both groups. Others have answered that greater productivity and growth coming from better trade and sectoral policies should help generate employment and income, given a setting of adequate overall economic policies and properly functioning markets and social institutions.

Small producers will also be helped by the disciplines that the URAA is bringing to subsidized and dumped exports, while it allows the implementation of a variety of programmes aimed at poor producers or consumers, including stocks for food security purposes and domestic food aid for populations in need. The issue here is the adequate design and funding of domestic policies to achieve the intended objectives of agricultural growth and poverty alleviation, which most certainly will not be helped by trade-distorting interventions either in developed or developing countries.

In general, low-income developing countries and LLDCs should emphasize to the international community the importance of creating and expanding a supportive international trade and financial environment and of implementing an integrated framework for economic and social development, with agricultural and trade policies being an integral part of the strategy. Appropriate measures would include—in addition to the agricultural trade issues suggested here—the continuation and enhancement of the reduction of the external debt of Heavily Indebted Poor Countries (the HIPC initiative) and the further liberalization of trade in textiles.

But improved international conditions should go hand-in-hand with a better domestic framework in developing and least-developed countries, including stable macroeconomic policies, open and effective markets, good governance, the rule of law, a vibrant civil society, and programmes and investments that expand opportunities for all, with special consideration for poor and disadvantaged groups.

Bringing Developing Countries into the Process

Developing countries, as small players in the global arena, should be interested and active participants in the design and implementation of international rules that limit the ability of larger countries to resort to unilateral action. Also, domestic legal and institutional frameworks in developing countries may be strengthened by the implementation of internationally negotiated rules that limit the scope for rent seeking and arbitrary projectionist measures. The developing countries as a group have much to gain from continued progress toward a transparent, rule-based, trading system in agriculture.

What are the requirements and skills for the developing countries to become effective members in the next WTO round? Any negotiation requires careful consideration of the legal, economic, and political dimensions that define the substance and possible evolution of the negotiations, as well as the diplomatic and negotiating techniques that may help in the attainment of the expected outcomes. Questions that need to be addressed include:

- What are the economic and social consequences of different WTO scenarios (quantitative estimation of impacts)? Knowing the impacts of alternative scenarios is crucial if developing countries are to represent their interests in the negotiation process.
- What are the legal issues being discussed (definition of obligations exemptions, time frame, and so on)? Detailed knowledge of international trade law is crucial if developing countries are not to be "shortchanged." The devil is in the details.
- Looking at the political process, who are the main actors and their interest and what type of alliances may drive the negotiations? Negotiators must understand the political economy of their own country and of other countries in the WTO if they are to negotiate effectively.
- With these elements, an adequate diplomatic and negotiating strategy must be defined and implemented.

Developing countries that have carefully considered all four components will be better prepared to participate effectively in the coming negotiations. Of course, limited financial and human resources act as an important constraint. However, developing countries may overcome some of the problems through collective action, for instance considering the creation of alliances with respect to their main export and import commodities and the markets they approach for their exports. An example is the Cairns Groups. This approach could reduce the fixed costs of negotiations., Spreading them over groups of countries, allow a better use of scarce technical expertise, and improve the bargaining position of developing countries. It could also be in the interest of the OECD countries to deal with negotiating blocs, which represent a smaller number of negotiating positions, rather than with numerous separate countries. The negotiations would be much more efficient and balanced.

13

The Future of Agricultural Trade

In the Uruguay Round, countries recognised that the long term solution for agriculture did not lie in administered prices, trade restrictions, supply controls, and export subsidies but rather in open, nondistorted markets. It is the time to take bold steps toward bringing agricultural trade into the 21st century by accelerating agricultural trade reform.

There are four key areas for accelerating reforms: eliminating export subsidies; increasing market access though substantial tariff cuts and expansion of tariff-rate quotas; cutting further trade-distorting domestic subsidies; and ensuring technical standards are based on sound science.

The world's farmers and ranchers are facing two difficult challenges at the dawn of the 21st century. First, they are being asked to provide more products at lower cost, higher quality, greater variety, and in a safer manner than ever demanded before. Second, they are being asked to produce this abundance on a shrinking natural resources base that is often subject to government regulations. Meeting these global challenges will require unleashing the production potential of world agriculture while practicing proper environmental stewardship. The ingenuity and hardwork we usually associate with farmers will be essential to meet these challenges, but they will not be sufficient unless we further reform agricultural, trade to create an environment that rewards risk and investment and encourages efficiencies.

Today's Agricultural Challenges

Farmers are responsible for feeding a rapidly growing world population. And despite progress over the years, too many people still are not getting enough food. Many countries including the United States, are working vigorously to promote technological innovations to meet the need for food and fiber in the coming years. However, as important as this work is, it is only part of the solution. These technologies and the hard work of the world's farmers need a trading environment that encourages investment and efficient production, and generates economic growth to finance production and consumption needs long-term trends in agriculture pose serious challenges for all farmers. The same technological advances that increase yields may result in lower prices. Increasing social concerns about effect of agricultural production on the environment ad living conditions result in new restrictions on farm activities. As urban dwellers and industry stake competing claims for land, water, and energy, many producers find their ability to farm made ever more difficult.

Two approaches to organizing the agricultural economy present a stark contrast in dealing with these challenges. One model, popular in Europe and Asia, is to retain an inward-looking agricultural system focused on supply control and government regulation geared to keeping farm prices high and, since guaranteed high prices are a drain on the treasury, to controlling production. Under this approach, bureaucrats try to assess the optimal level of national production—not so little that imports are needed and not so much that excess production; must be bought at high prices and; then dumped on world markets. This "command-and-control" structure stifles farmer efficiency and ingenuity and distorts world markets, especially as subsidized surpluses are regularly exported; and it does not address the challenge to farmers to produce food for the next century. It also ignores the interest of domestic consumers (who have to pay high internal prices) and producers in other countries (who have to compete with subsidized products). Of biggest concern is that the anti-market policies of this approach hamstring the agriculture sector from pursuing the technological advances needed to meet its future challenges.

Another approach is to place agriculture on a more market-oriented basis, particularly by removing trade barriers and reducing trade-distorting policies. Greater market orientation was the principle that actions agreed to in the last set of multilateral trade negotiations. In the Uruguay Round, countries recognized that the long-term solution for agriculture did not lie in administered prices, trade restrictions, supply controls, and export subsidies but rather in open, nondistorted markets. Now is the time to take bold steps towards bringing agricultural trade into the 21st century by accelerating agricultural trade reform.

The Gains from Trade

The benefit from free and fair trading of agricultural products have immediate effects on people. Eliminating trade barriers and reducing unfair competition will help ensure that farmers have incentives to produce and consumers have access to the products they desire. Liberalizing agricultural trade will contribute to better resource allocation by farmers, which has conservation benefits, rewards low-cost producers, encourages efficiencies, and removes the drag on economic growth.

Opening trading opportunities also increases the food security of food-importing countries by giving supplier countries the confidence required to put more land into production and to create marketing relationships. Trade provides consumers with year-round access to a greater variety of less expensive products, while rewarding producers who are able to find and meet specific consumer demands for high-value products. In a broader context, by allowing imports that are more efficiently produced elsewhere, trade encourages specialization in efficient agricultural and nonagricultural production.

More dramatically, trade literally saves lives. Without the international flow of food products from areas with abundant production to areas where food is scarce, many people in the world would be eating less or not at all. Trade has dynamic effects, as well, that push long-term productivity growth. For example, access to customers in overseas markets creates an incentive for technological innovation, resulting in exciting developments in improved seed varieties and production techniques. International markets also expand market outlets, raising prices and giving producers increased confidence to produce more than required merely for national needs, allowing productive farmers to not only feed their neighbours but literally feed the world.

Equally important, trade in agricultural products is becoming increasingly critical to farm and ranch incomes. Increased productivity and often times flat domestic demand increases the importance of reliable international markets. Foreign markets are not just a dumping ground for surplus products; overseas consumers value choice and quality, particularly when producers in their own country cannot meet their demands or when they are charged inflated prices. Consequently foreign and value-added agricultural producers, raising farm-gate prices and helping support the range of agriculture-related industries.

Political reality also encourages a focus on international markets: policies based on high government guaranteed prices are ultimately politically untenable because they are hugely expensive, unresponsive to the needs of customers and producers, insensitive to environmental and agronomic realities, and a shameful waste of economic assets. Rather than farming government programmes, our producers are looking for customers around the world.

While agricultural trade benefits consumers and producers alike, it is an area in which progressive reform is ardently opposed by entrenched domestic interests. Producers in some countries, cosseted by high guaranteed prices and protective tariffs, oppose any move toward greater market orientation. Intervention in the agricultural economy—measured by the Organization for Economic Cooperation and Development by summing price supports, direct payments, and other support as a per cent of total agricultural production—has actually increased in some countries from the levels at the beginning of the Uruguay Round. In the last set of multilateral trade negotiations, countries began the process of dismantling protection and delinking farm support from production decisions. Consequently, reforms have been undertaken by some countries.

The WTO Opportunity

The major objective in the upcoming farm talks is to accelerate the reform process initiated in the Uruguay Round. That means further substantial negotiations on tariffs, subsidies, and other trade-distorting measures so that the level and other trade-distorting measures so that the level and direction of trade are determined by market forces, not government intervention. *Four key areas are outlined below.*

(i) ***Export Competition:*** Export subsidies are the most distorting trade tool because the level and direction of trade is directly determined by government subsidies. Today, the European Union (EU) is the only substantial export subsidizer—nearly all other countries agreed not to use, or have only limited resourse to use, export subsidies in the last round of negotiations. EU farmers, responding to domestic prices frequently twice the world price, produce more products than can be consumed in Europe, but at such high prices that they can be sold abroad only with generous subsidies. These subsidies push other competitive suppliers out of the market (which is expensive and unfair) and discourage production in countries that have a comparative advantage in agricultural production (which is wasteful and is threatening both to the environment and to future farm production needs).

In the Uruguay Round negotiations, countries acknowledged the corrosive nature of subsidies and agreed to cap and reduce their use. The upcoming negotiations should eliminate them to ensure that countries do not resort to other policy tools that allow government spending to determine winners in the marketplace. Specifically, WTO members should look closely at curbing distorting state trading agricultural export monopolies that can disguise subsidies and exert distorting market power, along with other policies used to dispose of surplus commodities on a nonmarket basis.

(ii) ***Market Access:*** Measures applied at the border to stop trade currently are the principal barrier to a freer and more open trading environment for agriculture. Market access barriers deny efficient producers the chance to compete in other markets and limit the variety and quality of products available to consumers. Opening markets and maximizing trade opportunities are fundamental principles of WTO, and we still have a long way to go in agriculture to open markets to competition.

The Uruguay Round Agreement set agricultural trade on a more predictable basis by requiring that all nontariff measures, such as quotas and import bans, be converted to simple tariffs. While this was a necessary first step to removing trade barriers, many of the tariffs are still prohibitively high. For example, while the average tariff assessed by the United States on agricultural products is less than 5 per cent (and nearly zero for industrial products), the average agriculture tariff-rate quota (TRQ). Where only specific quantities of imports receive low duties. Many other commodities also; are subject to high tariffs.

As we start that next century, higher tariffs should not stop the flow of imported agricultural products. Where TRQs remain as a transitional step before we achieve more open trade, we expect more specific disciplines on the way in which they are administered. Similarly, we need to take a hard look at agricultural state trading monopoly. Importers; use of these state traders may have been justifiable when more restrictions allowed on farm trade, but in the tariff-only regime it is hard to see why a government needs to insert itself between an exports and an end-user.

(iii) ***Domestic Subsidies.*** Domestic subsidy programmes are often the root cause of other-distorting policies. Subsidy policies that increase domestic prices above world price levels can be maintained only if price-competitive imports are restricted. Additionally, overproduction generated by high domestic prices can be sold on world markets only with export subsidies that bring the price down to the world price. While reining in distortive domestic subsidy programmes has value in its own right for rationalizing agricultural production, the WTO negotiations will focus on their trade-distorting elements.

In the Uruguay Round negotiations, countries, agreed to distinguish trade-distorting subsidies (generally those linked to the production of a specific crop or related to price supports) from non-trade distorting subsidies (such as research and development, training and environmental production). The trade-distorting subsidies were capped, and the process of reducing allowable levels of subsidies began. This distinction is a good one: the nasty sort of subsidy that distorts markets and straitjackets producers should be cut, while programmes that will increase a country's ability to produce agricultural products in the next century without distorting production incentives should not be reduced.

(iv) ***Standards.*** As WTO members make progress on cutting tariffs and subsidies, the temptation increase to disguise trade barriers as health and safety measures or other innocuous-sounding "technical standards". Moreover, when regulations purportedly designed to protect health are instead vehicles for domestic protectionism, the credibility of the entire safety apparatus of a country is put up for questioning. When good science is replaced by politics, the basis for sound health policy is undermined. Therefore, increasing government accountability by putting the emphasis on sound science for health standards should discipline disguised barriers to trade and strengthen health policy.

In the Uruguay Round, countries agreed to a set of sound principles: each has the right to maintain health and safety measures, but these must be based on sound science, backed by scientific evidence and an assessment of the risk, and be no more trade-restrictive than required to meet health goals. In practice, countries have found that these principles work well—bogus measures adopted without scientific basis have been successfully challenged in the WTO without sacrificing health concerns. Creating a supportive environment for the propagation of yield-enhancing biotech products also is critical for meeting the needs of the coming century.

Agriculture is Different

Agriculture occupies a special place in the national economies of most countries around the world. Farmers are responsible for feeding and clothing people. Farming also holds a powerful claim on our national cultures that calls for the preservation of rural lifestyles and values. Farm production is subject to the cruel vagaries of weather and the relentless decline in prices and increases in costs. Some people point to these factors as justifying a different treatment for agriculture in the international economy, including justifying trade-distorting agricultural policies. This is wrong-headed; societies can support farms and preserve rural communities in ways that foster choice, protect natural resources, and expand trade.

Farm production in the next century cannot afford to be trapped in a static system in which prices are determined by government mandate, production decisions are controlled by central planners, and farmers are forced to produce only for local consumers. This myopic system cannot be sustained in any important agriculture producing society. Moreover, this type of system will not meet the needs of the coming century, when we will face unprecedented consumer demand and natural resource constraints.

Instead, I look forward to dynamic world of agricultural trade in which producers, exporters, and retailers apply the creativity of the human mind to the natural bounty of the earth. In this "new" world, we will produce a greater amount and variety of food than ever before, feed the coming billions, sustain our environment, and unlock economic resources otherwise stifled by moribund protectionism, ultimately raising living standards around the world.

14

Why Don't We Stop Tuberculosis?

Tuberculosis, a disease many people associate with sequestered sanatoriums that were long ago abandoned or razed, has now reemerged as the number one killer among the infectious or communicable diseases. The current TB epidemic is expected to grow worse, especially in India, because of the evolution of multi-drug-resistant strains and the emergence of AIDS, which compromises human immune systems and makes them more susceptible to infectious diseases.

The resurgence of tuberculosis comes at a time when other infectious diseases that were once thought to be well-controlled—malaria and cholera, among them—have increased and new diseases, notably AIDS, have emerged. Despite the advances in modern medicine, infectious diseases have persisted and continue to have a major effect on public health; in the 50 years following the discovery of antibiotics, efforts to control age-old epidemics have been overcome not by a lack of medical knowledge but by structural problems including the lack of adequate health care in many parts of India, and increased rates of travel and migration.

Tuberculosis has special characteristics that set it apart from other infectious diseases, most of which rely on mosquitoes, rats, or water to transmit infection. Tubercle bacilli only live in human tissues, and tuberculosis can only be transmitted by close contact with an infected person. In a healthy individual, the immune system is normally able to wall of and isolate the bacilli in a nodule. This essentially neutralizes the tubercle bacillus, so the person has what is referred to as an inert infection. If the immune system remains strong, there is only a 5 to 10 per cent chance of developing TB from an inert infection. But if the immune system is under severe stress—from HIV, diabetes, or chemotherapy for cancer, for example—the chances that the infection will develop into disease increase to as much as 10 per cent in a single year.

A person who has active TB can spread the infection simply by coughing, sneezing, singing, or even talking. Another person has only to inhale the bacilli to become infected. If the infection is not detected and treated promptly, one person with active tuberculosis can infect an average of 10 to 14 people in one year and sometimes many more.

Inert TB infections may show no symptoms at all. Only if those infections are activated will these people be at risk of developing the disease and transmitting it to others. Unfortunately, little is known about what activates a latent TB infection beyond the fact that people with healthy immune systems run a lows risk of developing an active case of TB.

Because the already poor and disenfranchised Indian Population carry a disproportionate burden of tuberculosis, the disease has a certain stigma attached to it. But the unsanitary and crowded living conditions that are often connected to poverty do not cause TB to spread; they increase the chances that the infection will spread from person to person and the chances that a person's immune system may already be weak and therefore less able to fight the infection. Despite the misconceptions, tuberculosis is exacerbated only by the failure to detect and treat the infection properly and by close contact with infected individuals.

More than 95 per cent of TB cases reported in 1995 were in the developing world, an estimated two-thirds of them in Asia. India accounted for 2.1 million cases. India is with a disproportionate number of cases because AIDS is spreading quickly, health services are inadequate, and little money is available for treatment.

To identify and diagnose TB must be combined with sufficient infrastructure and resources, such as vaccines, medicines, trained health personnel, and clinics. As with other diseases, funding for research and prevention and treatment programmes is essential. Thanks to modern medicine, there is a low-cost, effective TB treatment with high cure rates among infected adults. But if patients don't take the drugs consistently or don't complete treatment, TB strains develop that are more resistant to medicine, and sometimes even untreatable. If this drug regimen were used throughout India. It would reduce the rate of transmission and cut the number of deaths by half over the next 10 years.

The growing TB epidemic is a classic case of a public health crisis in India that could be headed off easily and inexpensively. Its fate will largely depend on the willingness of government and public health officials to invest up front in prevention and early intervention. If we ignore the extraordinary opportunity that exists now to fight the epidemic, we will pay a high price in lives and extensive health care costs later.

15

Children's Health and the Environment

Children today live in an environment vastly different from that of a few generations ago. Economic development, increased urbanisation and the consequences of war in many countries have added to the traditional environmental hazards, those problems associated with environmental pollution. Thus, while some traditional children's diseases such as diarrhoea, malnutrition and infectious diseases persist in many countries, environmentally-related illnesses such as asthma, respiratory illnesses due to environmental tobacco smoke (ETS), as well as mortality and morbidity due to injuries, are increasing. In childhood cancer in some countries and the potential risks of endocrine-disrupting chemicals are among the emerging health threats that need careful vigilance. Children of lower socio-economic status are likely to suffer disproportionately from all these health threats as a consequence of living in highly polluted environments, poor quality housing, lower levels of education, and of restricted access to environmental and health care services.

Children's Vulnerability

The concern for children's vulnerability to environmental health threats is based on several factors. Children receive greater exposures than adults do because they drink more water, eat more food and have higher breathing rates per unit of body weight. Because they are undergoing rapid growth and development, toxicant effects at specific times may have irreversible consequences. For example, if vital connections between nerve cells fail to form during brain development, there is high risk that the resulting neurobehavioural dysfunction will be permanent and irreversible. Also, because most children have more future years of life than adults, they have more time to develop any chronic disease that may be triggered by early environmental exposures.

Public Health Threats

Asthma, injuries, and the effects of environmental tobacco smoke (ETS) are among the most significant public health threats to children. Childhood asthma is increasingly prevalent in all most all countries. What causes asthma is not known, but several environmental factors, such as indoor air quality (particularly exposure to the house-dust mite) and ETS, have been linked with the increase in asthma. In addition, outdoor air pollutants such as particulates, sulphur dioxide and ozone can exacerbate asthma symptoms. ETS, especially smoking by the mother, is a known risk factor for asthma. ETS is also known to cause acute and chronic middle ear disease and is associated with sudden infant death syndrome (SIDS).

Potential for Prevention

The variation in asthma and injury rates and the evidence of the role of certain environmental factors underline the potential for prevention. Public policies should seek to avoid preventable childhood diseases by preventing exposures to environmental agents and considering children's characteristics and susceptibilities in the development of environmental health legislation. Promoting citizen awareness and participation in policy-making through education and access to environmental information are important elements in achieving a safe environment for children. In this context, children are not only consumers with rights, but also citizens who can play an active role towards their own protection.

International Awareness

Several international agreements have acknowledged children's vulnerabilities and have committed their signatories to protect children's health from the effects of a deteriorating environment. This year, many countries will address several of the environmental health threats to children through international and national action. It is expected that a large international collaborative initiative will result under the guidance of WHO and other international organisations.

16

Towards Healthy Cities

More than a third of the urban population in developing world live in housing of such poor quality with such inadequate provision for water, sanitation, drainage, garbage collection and health care that their health is constantly under threat. But, properly planned, cities can be safe and healthy.

In the cities of India, it is common for one child in three to die before the age of five and for virtually all infants, children and adults who survive to have disease burdens many times higher than they should.

Diarrhoea, tuberculosis and respiratory infections (each among the largest causes of death) are generally much increased by over-crowding. Many accidental injuries happen when there are three or more persons living in each small room in shelters made of flammable materials and there is little chance of providing occupants (especially children) with protection from open fires or stoves.

But cities also include some of the India's safest and most healthy neighbourhoods. High densities allow much lower costs for supplying each household with piped, treated water supplies and most forms of health, educational and emergency services.

Sanitation and drainage may be costly in cities, as complex systems are needed to cope with high densities and large population concentrations but city households can generally afford to pay more—and are prepared to do so if they get a good service.

Cities may be considered ecologically unsustainable because of high consumption and waste levels but well planned and managed cities can combine high living standards with remarkably low levels of energy consumption, resource use and wastes. The concentration of people and production creates many more possibilities of collecting and recycling wastes and for walking, bicycling and a high quality public transport.

For many, city-life is one of excessive work loads and drudgery, yet cities remain centres of culture-including the visual and decorative arts, music, dance, theatre and literature. Most cities have a large reserve of young people on whose initiative and energy they could draw to improve conditions—yet most such people find that their cities offer them little hope and little prospect of employment. If cities have such potential to provide healthy, stimulating and valued places to live and work for all age groups, why do so few achieve this?

Supporting Change

Much of the explanation is the lack of 'good governance'. Good governance in any city means encouragement and support from all levels of government for a great range of investments of capital, expertise and time by individuals, households, communities, voluntary organizations and NGOs-as well as private enterprises. In most cities in India, the total value of investments made by people in their own homes and neighbourhoods exceeds many times the total value of capital investments made by city and municipal authorities. Yet governments and aid agencies usually ignore (or deem illegal) most such efforts.

Most households who want their own home cannot afford to purchase one—or at least one that is legal. They cannot obtain housing loans so the cost of the house purchase can be spread over a number of years—as they cannot meet the (usually) inappropriate conditions set by banks or housing finance institutions. If they turn to building their own home-as most do—they have to occupy or purchase the site illegally. They often have to build on dangerous sites—in floodplains or on slopes with frequent landslides or mudslides—as the cost of safer sites is too high.

Even if they can qualify, for a housing loan, most such loans are for finished houses, not for incremental construction. And even when they have developed their own home and neighbourhood into a viable residential area, governments usually, refuse to provide these with roads, water supplies, drains and other essential infrastructure, because they are 'illegal'.

What would cities look like today if governments had supported these individual and community efforts by ensuring that land, building materials, credit and technical advice were as cheap and readily available as possible? Or if government-community partnerships had been formed to, at least, improve water supply, sanitation, drainage and health care.

These work within what is often called the 'social economic'—the great variety of initiatives and actions that are organized and controlled locally and that are not profit-oriented. The social economy includes the work of citizen groups, residents' associations, street or barrio clubs, youth clubs, and parent associations that support local schools. It includes many voluntary groups that provide services for the elderly, the physically disabled or other individuals in need of social. It often includes many initiatives that make cities safer and more fun-helping provide supervised play space, sport and recreational opportunities for children and youth. It may provide formal or informal supervision or maintenance of parks, squares and other public spaces.

The social economy not only 'gets things done' but also creates a dense fabric of relationships that allows citizens to work together in identifying and acting on local problems. Its value to a 'healthy city' is enormous, even if it is often forgotten by governments and international agencies.

The capacity of city authorities to govern is not the same as the capacity to invest, since these authorities can do much to encourage and support the social economy. City authorities can often greatly increase the supply and reduce the cost of land for housing by changing inappropriate regulations, streamlining planning and land use control, procedures and making better use of publicly owned land.

City authorities should also have the main role in enforcing legislation on, air and water pollution and occupational health and safety. This does not require large investments by public authorities, but it can do much to improve health and the quality of life in a city. Good governance also means managing competing claims and finding common ground between enterprises, trade unions and residents about what should be done to make the city more healthy.

Achieving a healthy city needs a representative political system through which the priorities of citizens and businesses can influence policies and actions. Democratic structures remain among the best checks on the misallocation of resources by city and municipal governments. Actively involving a wide range of local groups in developing 'city governance' helps ensure that the different priorities of a wide range of groups are addressed.

The key issue is not so much identifying what should be done to achieve more healthy cities. This is well known. It is identifying how it should be done, especially how governments and international agencies can support a vast range of activities by individuals, households and communities that help build and maintain healthy cities—which to date they have ignored or even (for many governments) repressed.

17

Health Care Relief in Conflict Situations

What Can we Learn from the Food Relief Experience?

Conflicts and war occur in many of the poorest nations where populations already suffer from severe ill-health. War leads to an increase in disease and to a worsening of the already fragile condition of populations. Health care itself becomes a victim of conflict. Many deaths which occur during these emergencies are not discretely related to the conflict itself but are the result of lacking access to public health services. Furthermore, conflict itself but are the result of lacking access to public health services. Furthermore, conflict contributes to the deterioration of already pre-existing structural weaknesses of the health care system. An example is the period of internal conflict in Uganda (1970-1986) when health services declined in the aftermath of the war due to the impact of foreign assistance and the planning vacuum in which the activities took place.

The Impact of Conflict on Health Care

Conflict and civil strife may lead to a major disruption of health services. This is not only a result of physical destruction but also of finding shortages since national governments increase spending on military activities. Casualties increase the demand for curative services which can divert already limited resources from preventive care.

In the case of the Sudanese civil war a large majority of health professionals was forced to abandon rural health services and left for urban areas or neighbouring countries in order to find new employment. Entire preventive health services such as immunization as well as water and sanitation projects collapsed leaving the population exposed to infectious diseases and epidemics. In urban areas, the gap in public health care provision is sometimes filled with the expansion of private services. In rural areas, private sector involvement in health care is rather marginal, apart from some omission hospitals or pharmacies. Therefore the non-formal health care sector often makes a substantial contribution towards health care.

With the rise of internal conflicts in Africa, more people suffer from emergency situations. This also increases the influence and impact of international donors. External assistance nowadays accounts for more than 25 per cent of government health expenditure in sub-Saharan Africa.

The size of donor involvement reflects the power of international agencies to control the policy domaine. Countries in conflict or post-conflict situations are under pressure to 'rescue' their health systems and accept global policies in exchange for aid assistance and relief.

However, in the period after 1991, donor organisations tended to increase their expenditures for high profile humanitarian operations rather than ordinary development activities. This shift may reflect the increasing influence of media covering some of the conflicts. Too often, organizations intervene with ad-hoc assistance without sufficient consultation at local level.

Donors' Perceptions in Designing Relief Interventions

Today, in many parts of sub-Saharan Africa development assistance has virtually collapsed and has been substituted by relief assistance. The problem is that relief interventions are based on a Western construction of reality, reflecting what is desirable and necessary in times of conflict. Most interventions therefore stress physical and material needs, presuming that the social aspect of food and health is not an immediate issue to address.

The question which arises here is on who's views and perceptions these needs are based? While donors interests may be guided from the perspective of ill-health, the recipient government may be concerned with the collapse of the economy. However, any intervention needs to take into account that local knowledge and practices are shaped by state interests as well as power relationships. The common belief that health care systems always collapse due to conflict is sometimes mistaken, considering the fact that today's internal conflicts are often fragmented, conflicts do not necessarily result in a breakdown of the health care delivery system.

Donors tend to respond with a 'package' approach and developing countries ministries of health increasingly play a symbolic role. The evidence suggests that international organizations tend to create verticle programmes which undermine national public health programmes. Foreign interventions are technically sophisticated and reorienting health are towards a more curative approach. Too little attentions given to strengthen the health care system within its own limits, providing more appropriate technology, drugs and emphasizing the training of local health staff.

Another vital issue concerns the existence of already fragile health information systems. Agencies tend to bring their own systems which leads to further fragmentation. The local perspective on what are the 'basic needs' in physical and social health are usually not considered. Health relief interventions do not recognize the potential of the communities and the non-formal health sector such as healers and traditional midwifes in supporting and maintaining health care sector presents a substantial contribution towards health. It is not the question between choosing either allopathic or traditional services, it is more the decision which kind of illness will be best treated by which practitioner. There is a need in further exploring the role of this sector particularly since this is sometimes the only service available for certain populations.

Responding to Local Needs

More community-based public health interventions could be vital to reduce mortality and morbidity. For example in Somalia during the 1992 war and famine high mortality rates due to measles and diarrhoea could have been prevented by involving the communities in primary health care activities such as immunization and nutrition improvement.

In the African context Tigray is an example where health services had been sustained and partially expanded during the civil war against the Ethiopian government. Local government structures called baitos promoting social and economic development. Baitos encouraged communities to establish revolving funds for drugs and medical equipment. It actually functioned as an early type of community financing system.

As mentioned above, the challenge in changing health care relief strategies is to overcome the approach of short-term interventions, particularly in a changing conflict environment where conflicts are complex and interruptions are no longer short-term. Therefore interventions need to be linked with the process of conflict resolution to avoid health care or food aid being used by politically dominant groups.

Food Relief in Conflict Situations

Food interventions have both a survival and a production function. For example, food-for-work may be part of an income programme or food aid can be monetized to generate local currency. However, food aids has to be seen beyond the objective to fulfil nutritional goals, it also defines relationships between social groups in regard to food accessibility and how food is shared. Food aid is aiming to meet people's basic food requirements and minimising risk and severity of disease by complementing services such as basic health care.

In more stable political conditions where free food aid is given it presents an income transfer by releasing income which normally is spent on food. However, in conflict situations food relief frequently becomes part of the dynamics of conflict such in the case of Sudan where it is used to sustain the struggle between the North and the South without resolving it. Furthermore, the military attack food supplies in the fight against rebels who depend on the support from the communities.

Health is also a matter of food security. When food insecurity coincides with conflict situations, health and survival are threatened. Food security provides some concepts on how and why vulnerable households manage to survive in periods of hardship (coping strategies).

Coping Strategies in African Trouble Zones

Today, most conflicts in Africa such as the one in the Great Lake Region, Angola or Congo cause major problems of food insecurity. They are linked to the civil wars which produce substantial social disruption as a result of massive population movements. The analysis of coping strategies showed that household respond to these conflict situations by eating less, selling livestock and land, or trying to find new sources of income.

In some emergency situations, however, such coping mechanisms may fail. In the case of the war in Mozambique food aid was vital since coping strategies were limited and people had to sell all their assets which was particular true for internationally displaced persons and refugees.

It has been argued that food relief by passes local structures in favour of those qualifying on a nutrition status criterion, decided by international organizations, or it may attract populations to refugee camps to receive free food rations and thereby undermines local production. In the case of Rwanda food aid was targeted at the internally displaced and left out the local population. This can be due to donor bias in needs assessment.

Food scarcity is not always so result of civil war but its creation may be rather a political objective. An example is food relief manipulated by local elites and the military like in the case of Sudan. It can be summarized that generally relief operations often bear the risk of fuelling the process of instability and violence rather than helping to contain the situation.

Lessons from Food Relief for the Health Sector?

Through the experience of food relief in recent civil wars such as Sudan, Somalia, Mozambique etc., there has been an increasing awareness of the economic and political context in which operations take place. Like food relief, health care is a political tool which can, if not properly targeted, undermine peoples access to health care services. While food production is linked to food security, it is more difficult to identify factors leading to self-sufficiency in health care.

As mentioned above, food aid is aiming to insure survival. It also has an economic aspect, protecting household assets. Health care relief is targeted to assure immediate physical survival based on the importance of social health. Unfortunately, curative interventions hardly consider the socio-cultural dimension of health. Therefore it would be beneficial if health care interventions consider local norms and traditions. Interventions should be compatible and complement local health programmes. The emphasis should be on strengthening formal and non-formal health institutions both in service provision and training.

In food relief, distribution and needs assessment identification are controversial issues for discussion. While the programme design is shaped by donors perceptions, the actual programmes are influenced by the priorities of some powerful leaders as well as the socio-economic and political context.

Health care interventions need to analyse these issues in the context of economic and political systems in order to identify the most vulnerable groups, for example populations living in areas which are more, operations require a stronger involvement of communities both as users and active participants to carry out and maintain public health programmes.

There is a need for a new concept to be designed which applies to chronic emergencies. In the absence of a policy framework, guidelines need to be developed in order to overcome the inconsistency in planning and implementation. Donors need to change their assumptions on which they plan their health relief responses. A starting point in improving the efficiency of these operations is to provide institutional support to local authorities and organisations and involve them in the planning and implementation of programmes.

18

The Environment, the Economy and Public Health—An Integrated View

The environment is central to the health of people and their economies. Just as a foetus is totally dependent on the life-support system of the mother during her pregnancy, so the health and vitality of people and their economies are totally dependent on their environments. Unfortunately, many people do not see it that way. They either see the environment as dependent on the economy—such as the politician who says: "let's make the economy strong, then we'll fix the environment when we can afford it"—or they see little connection between health and the environment, whether they are "deep greens" campaigning on ecological issues or doctors treating individual patients and individual illnesses. Whether we are politicians, greens or doctors, is there not a more efficient way to fulfil our aims? For this, a broader perspective is essential.

All economies are sub-systems of the larger environmental system which provides the:

- Sources of energy and materials;
- Sinks for pollution and other wastes;
- Services of water, nutrients and carbon recycling.
- Space for living, working and aesthetics ("a walk in the woods and the song of a bird")

Neglect of this life-support system of the "4 S's" leads to weaker or defunct economies as vegetation, food, soils, water or air become contaminated or exhausted and gradually fail to support economic activity. This is dramatically illustrated in the Aral Sea region, or the collapsed Canadian salmon fishing communities.

Indirect Social Costs

Less catastrophic but still costly is where economic damage is caused by pesticides and nutrient contamination of groundwater, involving millions of Rurpees in water treatment. This is a social cost to the economy that the agricultural sector does not include in the price of its food: an economic distortion that reduces the real wealth of society via false price signals that encourage the over -use of pesticides and fertilisers. Similarly, the "external" costs on society of road-respiratory-induced accidents, noise, respiratory and circulatory diseases and congestion amount to a lot of money to any government but these costs are not borne by transport users, which mean that transport is encouraged beyond the level that is economic for society as a whole. By internalising these externalities via taxes and other means, the market prices for transport would become fairer and more efficient. Currently only about 30 per cent of transport externalities are covered by transport taxes. But if the health of an economy is dependent on the health of its environment, what about the health of its people?

Without access to the basics of clean water, shelter, fresh air and food, people obviously suffer. Even in more developed economies where the link between everyday life and the environment is not so visible, the role of environmental factors in disease and well-being is significant. Most of the major diseases such as heart disease, cancer, respiratory diseases and allergies have an environmental as well as a genetic component within a multi-factorial chain of causation. And while each environmental factor may be small, if the links in the chain of causation are inter-dependant, as they often appear to be then removing even a small link can break the chain.

Environmental Factors

Take asthma in children, for example. There seem to be many causes, from a child's genetic inheritance to its nutritional status, which in turn help determine how it reacts to the many environmental factors, both indoor (such as mites, pets, damp, environmental tobacco smoke, nitrogen oxides) and outdoor (such as pollen and pollution from industry and traffic), that have been implicated in asthma causation. Therefore it is clear that diagnoses of asthma and many other diseases should systematically embrace environmental factors. This will be a significant challenge for doctors whose time is scarce and whose training is not usually appropriate.

This multi-causal chain will vary in its exact make-up from child to child, but for children overall, even if the environmental factors such as damp housing or traffic fumes may be less important than, say, genetic make-up or nutritional status, the environmental factors may be the ones that can be most cost effectively removed, thus breaking the casual chain. And, as with many environmental issues, there are secondary benefits of action, such as less noise or fewer accidents from traffic reduction, or energy savings from dry houses, which further justify the environmental actions even where exact causations are not well understood.

The environmental causes of disease and ill health are a controversial and ill understood area of science and opinions vary about their significance. Some say that, for Western Europe, perhaps 2-3 per cent of public disease and ill-health is determined by known environmental factors but others maintain that it must be far more significant. They point to the sharp increase over the last two or three decades in asthma, allergies, and cancers (particularly of the reproductive organs such as breast and testicles) and related ill-health such as sperm count decline, which cannot be explained by genetic causes. They also observe that the large differences in health between the socio-economic classes cannot be explained without involving significant environmental causation.

It is thought that the ubiquitous presence of low doses of mixtures of chemicals in food, drink, air, consumer products and the general environment are playing some role in public ill health, even if the evidence for this is far from substantial.

Impact on Public Health

But what about environmental programmes and campaigns being little concerned with health? Well, history so far shows that the environment only gets serious attention when it is seen to be damaging either the economy or public health. Yet because "everything connects" in "socio-enviro" systems, action to stop infectious diseases from water contamination, or to reduce skin cancer from ozone depletion, leads to a better environment for all species. And if upland forests are preserved because they are seen to be cheaper and more effective water regulators (which reduce the risk of lowland flooding) than dams, then upland biodiversity benefits anyway, even if it was last in the queue for political attention.

Although public health may be seen by some as only a small part of "the environment", much environmental progress depends upon the political weight of the health impacts. For example, the cost benefit exercise on the current multi-pollutant/effect programme on acidification, eutrophication and low-level ozone shows that it is the benefits to human health, not eco-system damage, that provide the main economic justification for further reductions in SO_2, NO_2 and NH_3. Ecologists need the language of public health in order to maximise political support for the environment. So, it is out of our specialist "boxes" of economics, health and ecology, and into a shared systems approach, with integrated programmes that build partnerships for progress.

19

Action for Safe Motherhood

Countries vary enormously in terms of the situations and challenges they face and their capacity to address these. However, experience from around the world over the past decade has demonstrated that a number of features are common to successful efforts to address maternal mortality. Reducing maternal mortality requires coordinated, long-term efforts. Actions are needed within families and communities, in society as a whole, in health systems, and at the level of national legislation and policy. Further, interactions among the interventions in these areas are critical to reducing maternal morality and to building and supporting momentum for change.

Legislative and Policy Actions

Changes in legislation and policy are essential to ensure safe motherhood. Long-term political commitment is an essential prerequisite. When decision-makers at the highest levels are resolved to address maternal mortality, the resources needed will be mobilized and the essential policy decisions will be taken. Without this level of commitment over the long term projects cannot become programmes and activities cannot be sustained.

A supportive social, economic, and legislative environment allows women to overcome the various obstacles that limit their access to health care, such as distance from their homes to appropriate health facilities, lack of transport and, more critically, financial and social barriers. Proper maternal health care is limited when women have to pay for services and essential drugs, and when they must bear substantial hidden costs such as time lost for housework, paid employment, food production, and child care. Legislation that supports women's access to care must be formulated to permit health workers at the periphery of the health system to perform specific life-saving functions. Failing this, only highly skilled health professionals, based largely in urban centres, can provide such care, and only women with sufficient money and the means to reach such centres can benefit from it.

With these objectives, careful review of national laws and policies is necessary, particularly in the following areas:

- ***Family Planning.*** Statutes that restrict women's access to family planning services (e.g. by requiring that a woman be married or that she should have her husband's approval) should be repealed. Policies must ensure that all couples and individuals have access to good-quality, voluntary, client-oriented, and confidential family planning information and to services that offer a wide choice of effective contraceptive methods. Policies should address regulatory, social, economic, and cultural factors that limit women's control over sexuality and reproduction, in order that pregnancies that are too early, too late, or too frequent may be avoided.
- ***Adolescents and Children.*** Polices and programmes should encourage later marriage and childbearing and an expansion of the economic and educational opportunities for girls and women. Promotion of good nutrition in childhood and adolescence, as well as supplementation if necessary during pregnancy, provides protection for both women and their future children. Policies should also enable adolescents to take responsibility for and protect their sexual and reproductive health, and

facilitate their access to health information and services. All children, before they reach the age at which they become sexually active, need to be taught the risks of unprotected sex and helped to develop the skills needed to protect themselves from sexual coercion.

- ***Barriers to access.*** Assigning health workers trained in midwifery to village-based health facilities can help overcome problems of distance and transport. Health workers should also be trained to deal sympathetically with women patients. Policies should support the provision of services at minimum cost; at the same time, health workers should have job security, be paid adequate wages, and be provided with sufficient supplies to do their jobs. Policies that will increase women's decision-making power, particularly in regard to their own health, are also essential.

- ***Regulation of Practice.*** Protocols and statutes aimed at providing both routine maternal care and referral facilities for obstetric complications at each level of the health system need to be developed. Responsibilities at each level for supervision, deployment of health care personnel, remuneration, and reporting procedures must be defined nationally. Development and promotion of education and training curricula are important, as is the setting of national norms and standards to govern the selection of trainees, trainers, and supervisors.

- ***Delegation of Authority.*** Services should be decentralized so that facilities are available as close to people's homes as possible. Adequate supplies and equipment and trained staff should be available in all health facilities, particularly in rural and remote areas, together with written policies and protocols to guide service provision and to allow certain functions to be delegated to personnel at lower levels (when appropriately trained).

- ***Abortion.*** Availability of services for management of abortion complications and post-abortion care should be ensured by appropriate legislation. Where abortion is not prohibited by law, facilities for the safe termination of pregnancy should be made available. National policy can discourage unsafe abortion practices by promoting protection against unwanted pregnancy, and national health campaigns to publicize the risks of unsafe abortion and the need to recognize and seek treatment for abortion complications.

20

Safe Motherhood is a Human Rights Issue

The death of a woman during pregnancy or childbirth is not only a health issue but also a matter of social injustice. Of the human rights currently acknowledged in national constitutions and in regional and international human rights treaties, many can be applied to safe motherhood. Many such treaties and conventions are based on the 1948 Declaration of Human Rights (1) they include the Convention on the Elimination of All Forms of Discrimination against Women (2) the Convention on the Rights of the Child (3) the European Convention for the Protection of Human Rights and Fundamental Freedoms (4) the American Convention on Human Rights (5) and the African Charter on Human and Peoples' Rights (6).

Human rights of relevance to safe motherhood can be grouped into the following four principal categories:

- **Rights relating to life, liberty and security of the person,** which require governments to ensure both access to appropriate health care during pregnancy and childbirth, and women's rights to decide whether, when, and how often to bear children. Governments must therefore address factors within the economic, legal, social, and health systems that deny women these fundamental rights.

- **Rights relating to the foundation of families and of family life,** which require governments to provide access to health services and other facilities that women need to establish families and to enjoy life within a family.
- **Rights relating to health care and the benefits of scientific progress, including health information and education,** which require governments to provide access to good sexual and reproductive health care with appropriate referral systems. The measures need to ensure safe motherhood can be provided through primary health care irrespective of a country's level of economic development. Central to these rights is information on a range of reproductive health issues, including family planning, abortion, and sex education.
- **Right relating to equality and nondiscrimination,** which require governments to provide access to services such as education and health care without discriminatory grounds such as sex, marital status, age, and socioeconomic class. Discriminatory policies include requirements for a woman to obtain the consent of her husband for particular health care interventions, requirements for parental authorization which have a differential impact on girls, and laws that criminalize medical procedures that only women need. Governments are in violation of their obligations when they fail to implement laws that effectively protect women's interests or to allocate health resources to meet women's particular need for safe pregnancy and childbirth.

The actions that governments need to take to promote safe motherhood as a human right fall into three groups:

- **Reforms of laws** that prevent women from attaining the highest possible levels of health and nutrition needed for safe pregnancy and childbirth and that inhibit access to reproductive health information and services such as laws requiring women in need of health care to seek the authorization of husbands or other family members first.

- **Implemention of laws** that foster women's rights to good health and nutrition and that protect women's health interests such as laws that prohibit child marriage, female genital mutilation, rape, and sexual abuse. Every effort should be made to implement laws that encourage the healthy timing of births, such as those that support the education of girls, set a minimum age for marriage, and ensure women's access to essential health care.
- **Application of human rights** in national legislation and policy to advance safe motherhood.

21

The Nature and Causes of Drug Addiction

Man has been experimenting for thousands of years with a variety of naturally occurring substances that act on his nervous tissues: alcohol to intoxicate a weary mind, belladonna to calm an angry intestine or to poison an adversary, opium to overcome worry and strain. The relief of pain, in particular, in an age-old aim of mankind, and various narcotic and sleep-producing agents were probably used by primitive man. But for many men there is another kind of pain—the pain of being—and from time immemorial some men have been trying to expand their vision, enhance their appreciation of their world, change their mood, alter their inner existence, or stupefy their awareness with such drugs as alcohol, opium, and cannabis.

Drugs, chemical substances that affect the functions of living things, are used in treating, preventing, and diagnosing diseases. The most important source of drugs today is chemical synthesis. The increase in the manufacture of drugs has resulted in the development of 25,000 or more drugs and drug products. Many drugs are potentially dangerous chemicals that can cause serious, sometimes fatal, poisoning if used incorrectly: governments of various countries, therefore, have established certain legal requirements concerning drug use.

USES: The main purpose of the use of drugs is to cure disease or correct a disorder. Chemotherapeutic drugs, such as the antibiotics, the sulfa drugs, and the antimalarial drugs, flight infection by acting directly on disease-causing invading organisms, either immobilizing or killing them. Some chemotherapeutic drugs are also used to suppress or prevent infection.

Drug Toxicity

No drug is free of toxic effects. This factor is what ultimately limits the usefulness of drugs. Some of the untoward effects of drugs are trivial and can be readily tolerated. Others, however, are serious and may even be fatal. Some toxic effects of drugs are merely extensions of the drug's therapeutic effects.

This is why drugs never should be taken except under the guidance of a physician. A physician is aware of the potential hazards of a drug and is prepared to act promptly if toxicity occurs. Furthermore, the physician is aware that many of the toxic effects produced by drugs are unexpected, bizarre, and often not clearly related to the taking of a drug.

Many people suffer from drug allergy—one of the most serious problems of pharmacology. Penicillin, for example, is an extremely safe drug for most people, but it produces hypersensitivity reactions in about 15 per cent of the population. In some cases the reaction is so serious that it is necessary to forbid the future use of penicillin because of the risk of death. Drug allergy takes many different forms; skin reactions varying from a mild rash to severe dermatitis.

Drug Addiction and Abuse. It is very likely that every society has had mood-changing drug and that there have always been individuals who used them in ways that were not socially approved. In this sense, drug abuse, the socially nonsanctioned use of a drug, is universal and so old as history. Which behaviours are called drug abuse varies from culture to culture and from time to time within the same culture. Since laws do not always correspond to prevalent social attitudes, there may be times when users of an illegal drug are not considered to be drug abusers. From a pharmacological viewpoint, attitudes toward drugs are often inconsistent or irrational. Some drugs may be totally outlawed, while others with similar actions are made generally available and may be self-administered with full social approval.

The repeated use of some drugs can lead be a dependence on the drug, in which the effects of the drug or the conditions associated with its use are felt by the users to be necessary for their well-being. Dependence may vary in intensity from a mild inclination to a strong craving or compulsion to use the drug. Severe dependence may result in a type of behaviour is also known as Compulsive drug use, and since a severe dependence on any self-administered drug is generally not socially approved, the term is usually synonymous with compulsive drug abuse. One obvious exception is the use of tobacco, where social acceptance is so complete that even heavy compulsive use, which is damaging to the user's health, is commonly not considered to be drug abuse.

The term drug addiction has been defined in many ways, but in this article it is used to mean a behavioural pattern of compulsive drug use characterized by an overwhelming involvement with the procurement and use of the drug and the high tendency of the user to relapse to drug use after a period of abstinence. It is synonymous with intensive or severe drug dependence. Contrary to popular belief, drug addiction is not the same as physical dependence on a drug. Physical dependence is a physiological or biochemical condition produced by the administration of a drug to the extent that a characteristic pattern of signs and symptoms appears when the drug is withdrawn and disappears when the drug is administered again. Physical dependence can be produced by a wide variety of drugs that are used in everyday medical practice. Some drugs that produce physical dependence are not pleasant to take and are neither abused nor used compulsively. Also, not all withdrawal symptoms are associated with a craving for the drug that produced the physical dependence.

The Nature and Causes of Drug Addition

If opium were the only drug of abuse, and the only kind of abuse were one of habitual, compulsive use, discussion of addiction might be a simple matter. But opium is not the only drug of abuse, and there are probably as many kinds of abuse as there are drugs to abuse, or indeed, as may be there are persons who abuse. Various substances are used in so many different ways by so many different or one definition could possibly embrace all the medical, psychiatric, psychological, sociological, cultural, economic, religious, ethical, and legal considerations that have an important bearing on addiction. Prejudice and ignorance have led to the labelling of all use of nonsanctioned drugs as addiction and of all drugs, when misused, as narcotics. The continued practice of treating addiction as a single entity is dictated by custom and law, not by the facts of addiction.

Many substances are capable of acting on a biological systems, and whether a particular substance comes to be considered a drug depends, in large measure, upon whether it is capable of eliciting a "drug like" effect that is valued by the user. There is nothing intrinsic to the substances themselves that sets one active substance is imparted to it by use. Caffeine, nicotine, and alcohol are clearly drugs, and the habitual, excessive use of coffee, is not addiction. The same could be extended to cover tea, chocolates, or powered sugar, if society wished to use and consider them that way. The task of defining addiction, then is the task of being able to distinguish between opium and powdered sugar while at the same time being able to embrace the fact that both can be subject to abuse. This requires a frame of reference that recognizes that almost any substance can be considered a drug, that almost any drug is capable of abuse, that one kind of abuse may differ appreciably from another kind of abuse, and that the effect valued by the user will differ from one individual to the next for a particular drug, or from one drug to the next drug for a particular individual. This kind of reference would still leave unanswered various questions of availability, public sanction, and one kind of effect rather than another at a particular moment in history, but it does at least acknowledge that drug addiction is not a unitary condition.

Effects on the Mind and Body. The effects of drugs similar in many ways to those of alcohol. Low doses usually produce relaxation and decreased anxiety; higher doses produce drowsiness. Even if people can stay awake, they may appear confused and show poor judgement and loss of emotional control. Slurred speech, a staggering gait, muscular incoordination and nystagmus (rapid involuntary eye movements) are also characteristic effects. Although alcohol and the sedative-hypnotics are all depressants of the nervous system, low or moderate doses can produce an effect that resembles stimulation. The individual may become euphoric and more active, and show a decrease in inhibitions. Very high doses produce coma and death due to respiratory failure.

Drugs in Psychiatry. Drugs that are used either alone or in conjunction with psychotherapy to treat psychiatric illness. The medical treatment of psychiatric illness is based on a firm conviction that the patient's bahaviour is in fact a symptom of an illness and not simply a variant of acceptable behaviour in society. The study of drug effects on mental processes is called psycho pharmacology.

Certain patterns of disease with mental manifestations are biologically characteristic of humans. The use of drugs to treat these disease patterns is directed either at alleviating symptoms or at inhibiting or stopping the underlying disease processes. Diseases that have purely psychological causes, but appear in ways that disturb society or distress the individual, are often treated with nonspecific remedies, that either sedate or alert the individual. For all mental illness with specific biological causes, psychopharmacologists seek to develop drugs that change the biological functioning of the individual so that the symptoms of disease either do not occur or have a lesser impact on his or her life and behaviour.

The use of drugs in the treatment of psychiatric illness is not a denial of the importance of psychological or social factors in the causation or pattern of a disease. Drug treatment of psychiatric illness is based on the principle that the human nervous system is always a chemical biological system. Some psychiatric treatment systems—for example, psychoanalysis—do not utilize drug treatment. Some mental health experts feel that the use of drugs is only for the control of patients and not their treatment.

Social and Ethical Issues of Drug Use

Conflicting Values in Drug Use: The social and economic requirements of modern society may have undergone a radical change in the last few decades, even though the inertia of the existing social character, its desires and its values, will be felt for some time to come. In one major sense, current drug controversies are a reflection of this cultural lag with all of the consequent conflict of wishes and that result from the lack of good correspondence between traditional teachings and the view of the world as it is now being perceived by large numbers within society. Modern society is in a state of rapid transition, and this transition is not without its untoward consequences in terms of stability.

Cultural transitions notwithstanding, the dominant social order has strong negative feelings about any nonsanctioned use of drugs that contradicts its existing value system. Can society succeed if individuals are allowed unrestrained self-indulgence? Is it bad to rely on something so much that one cannot exist without it? Is it legitimate to take drugs if one is not sick? Does one have the right to decide for oneself what one needs? Does society have the right to punish someone if he has done no harm to himself or to others? These are difficult questions that do not admit to ready answers. One can guess what the answers would be to the nonsanctioned use of drugs. The traditional ethic dictates harsh responses to conduct that is "self-indulgent" or "abusive of pleasure". But how does one account for the quantities of the drugs being manufactured and consumed today by the general public? It is one thing to talk of the few hundred thousand or so "hard" narcotic users who are principally addicted to the opiates. One might still feel comfortable in disparaging the widespread illicit use of hallucinogenic substances; these are still the "other guys." But the sedatives, tranquilizers, sleeping remedies, stimulants, alcohol, coffee, tea, and tobacco are complications that trap the advocate in some glaring inconsistencies. It may be asked by partisans whether the cosmetic use of stimulants for weight control is any more legitimate than the use of stimulants to "get with it?"; whether the conflict-ridden businessman or the conflict-ridden housewife is any more entitled to relax chemically (alcohol, tranquilizers, sleeping aids, sedatives) than the conflict-ridden adolescent?"; Whether physical pain is any less bearable than mental pain or anguish? Billions of pills and capsules of a nonnarcotic type are manufactured yearly.

Sedatives and tranquilizers account for somewhere around 12 to 20 per cent of all doctor's prescriptions. In addition there are about 150 different sleeping aids that are available for sale without a prescription. The alcoholic beverage industry produces countless millions of gallons of wine and spirits and countless millions of barrels of beer each year. One might conclude that there is a whole drug culture; that the problem is not confined to the young, the poor, the disadvantaged, or even to the criminal that existing attitudes are at least inconsistent, possibly hypocritical. One always justifies one's own drug use, but one tends to view the other fellow who uses the same drugs as an abuser who is weak and undesirable. It must be recognized that the social consensus in regard to drug use and abuse is limited, conflict ridden, and often glaringly inconsistent. The problem is not one of insufficient facts but one of multiple objectives that at the present moment appear unreconcilable.

22

Link Between Disability and Poverty

Disability affects nearly every fifth household in developing countries and is a prevalent contributing factor to family poverty.

An already poor household has an added financial burden when a disabled family member is not involved in productive activities. In the context of extreme poverty, a disability may sometimes turn into an asset when the person uses begging as a way to bolster the family income. But this is a degrading path that does not lead out of poverty.

What aggravates the situation is the fact that poverty is identified as one of the main causes of disability. This is especially so for those at the lowest strata of society who live in precarious conditions without education, hygiene and health care.

An important element of measures aimed at families living in absolute poverty is that they learn how to prevent disability. They must also learn that a disabled family member can take part in economic activities.

Increasing the economic usefulness of a disabled household member can help to reduce the poverty of many families. The income earned by the disabled person not only benefits him or her but the entire household as well.

However, anti-poverty strategies which target disabled household members without attempting to alleviate general household poverty would likely be futile.

One widespread misconception is that disabled people are unable to earn a living and to be self-reliant. As a consequence, disabled people are often targeted only for passive measures of income replacement and social welfare schemes. Active measures in their favour are conceived of as social activities and not economically relevant. Such misconceptions generate and reinforce exclusion, which in turn perpetuates poverty.

This highlights a dimension of poverty often overlooked by economists. They define poverty only in terms of household income. But poverty also means to lack of social status and to lose human dignity.

Thus a basic criterion for an anti-poverty strategy at the micro-level is whether it serves to establish human dignity. An approach which merely dishes out state subsidies or international aid to the destitute keeps the recipients in a position of dependence.

Targeting specific groups for poverty alleviation measures is always a highly sensitive issue. It can damage the fragile social fabric and may result in greater poverty for some while favouring others. Such a risk may be avoided through a participatory approach which actively involves the poor and assists them in their efforts to gain control over their lives.

Disabled people are more likely to be poorer than their non-disabled peers because of the discrimination which accompanies disability, not because of the impairment itself.

They suffer from social exclusion and frequently find themselves trapped in a web of neglect. The problem is even more acute for disabled women, who encounter enormous prejudices and obstacles in their quest to participate in social and economic life.

A more enlightened society will seek to integrate disabled people, to give them opportunities to learn and to work as others do. It will adjust the physical environment to accommodate their special needs.

This planet belongs to all people. If some people are trapped somewhere, we must all come forward to remove the causes of their discomfort. At the same time we must leave our shores open for anybody who decides to join us, or anybody who decides to part our company.

Poverty denies a person control over his destiny. Poverty means not being able to tell what tomorrow would be like. If we examine the situation carefully we will see that the poverty is neighter created by the poor, nor sustained by the poor. It is the system of policies and institutions that we have built around us that creates and sustains poverty. Poverty is the denial of human rights. Over one billion people live below the absolute poverty line right now on this planet, are denied of almost all human rights. There is no way one can defend the existence of poverty anywhere. Poverty is a disgrace for the entire man-kind. Because we allow another humanbeing to die of hunger, or malnutrition, or common curable diseases, or exposure to climate, we are reduced to no less humanbeings. If a particular world system is responsible for creating this massive poverty we must act to replace it.

Resource-wise or technology-wise, there is no reason why poverty should exist and continue to deepen and widen. If we make up our minds to wipe out poverty from the surface of the earth, the worst aspect of poverty can be removed within the next couple of decades.

Each humanbeing is a wonderful creation of the creator. Each humanbeing is born with great potentials. Poverty denies any opportunity for a person to achieve any of his/her potential. We have built a world system which is in the habit of pushing people down not building them up. It creates barriers around individuals, rather than remove them.

The most effective step that we must take to remove poverty is to create a system which creates enabling conditions for people and removes the existing barriers. The institutional barriers were skilfully crafted over the centuries to benefit a handful of people.

Resource-poor nations with high incidence of poverty waste away enormous human capability each day by denying poor people the use of their energy and ingenuity. If they could have been made economically active, not only they could have contributed in the national production, they would have helped expand the domestic market for the products produced. The disabled one can be transformed into the engine of growth if we only allow them to unleash their capacity.

We cannot be at peace with ourselves if we know there is a humanbeing who lives a life worse than an animal. A humanbeing is supposed to live differrrently than an animal. He/she is supposed to live a life with human dignity. Human dignity is what distinguishes a humanbeing from an animal. When we cannot ensure this dignity for others, our own dignity becomes an empty pretence.

There must be a thousand and one ways to remove poverty from the earth. We may or may not know some of those ways already. Obviously there are many more ways yet to be designed, each more effectively than others. When we shall find them, how many of them we shall find, how quickly we find them, will depend on how eager we are to find them. But to say that poverty cannot be overcome, directly and quickly, is to underestimate the capacity of human mind.

23

Taking Poverty to Heart, Non–communicable Diseases and the Poor

Non-communicable Diseases (NCDs) are the leading cause of death worldwide. Their emergence as the predominant health problem in wealthy countries accompanied economic development. As a result, NCDs are often referred to as 'diseases of affluence'. But is this a misleading term? It suggests that these are not major problems for the world's poor, which is quite simply wrong, as this article illustrates. Is it time to rethink policy on NCDs?

NCDs include cardiovascular disease (CVD), such as stroke and hearth attack, diabetes, chronic lung disease, cancer, diseases of bones and joints, and mental illness. The single biggest killer is coronary heart disease, followed by other CVDs, cancer and chronic lung disease. Diabetes is a major contributor to deaths from CVD, but also causes its own unique complications. Common risk factors for these conditions include smoking, physical activity, obesity and diets high in saturated fat and sodium and low in fruit and vegetables.

By 2020, NCDs will be the biggest cause of death in all regions apart from sub-Saharan Africa. It is predicted that in 2010, the number of people with diabetes worldwide will be double the level in 1995 and that the biggest increase (both proportionately and in absolute number) will be in poorer regions. CVD occurs at an earlier age in developing countries, increasing the potential adverse economic and social consequences.

NCDs are already major health problems for adults in the poorest countries of the world. Demographic data show that age-specific death rates from NCDs in Tanzania are higher than in wealthier countries. Mortality rates for some NCDs, such as stroke, are particularly high. However, while NCDs account for 80 per cent of adult deaths in developed regions, the figure is less than 30 per cent in Tanzania, reflecting the continuing burden of infectious disease. Countries like Tanzania suffer the 'worst of both worlds'. Even within a country, 'diseases of affluence' is a misleading term. A more accurate label is 'diseases of Urbanisation'. Several studies from developing countries show increased levels of high blood pressure and other NCD risk factors in urban compared to rural populations. Even within urban areas, the more affluent do not always suffer the greatest burden.

The rise of NCDs in developing countries is inextricably linked to economic and cultural globalisation. This is exemplified by the activities of multinational tobacco companies. Tobacco-related deaths will exceed the toll due to HIV and become the single largest preventable cause of death by 2020. Curbing the effects of globalisation on the prevention and treatment of NCDs will also require regulation of food and agriculture multinationals and the pharmaceutical and healthcare industries.

Much of the projected rise in NCDs is preventable, particularly that due to smoking, poor diet, physical inactivity and obesity. Early action in some populations could prevent the emergence of these risk factors altogether; in other, the challenge is to reduce established levels. Although it is unclear whether all major risk factors are equally important in every region, the strength and consistency of data on the core risk factors in several ethnic groups justify preventative action now.

Lessons from risk factor intervention studies in rich and middle income countries suggest that success requires:

- Broad intersectoral action
- Community participation
- Appropriate legislation
- Involvement of appropriate NGOs
- Health services changes—to manage those at high risk and promote public education.

Even apparently minor changes, such as a small fall in average population blood pressure, can have substantial benefits. However, some preventative programmes have produced disappointing results and almost all have failed to halt the ubiquitous increase in obesity. This highlights the difficulty of promoting healthy behaviour by individuals who are surrounded by barriers to change and inducements to lead an unhealthy lifestyle.

Health systems in developing countries face both a growing need for prevention programmes and increasing numbers of individuals requiring treatment. The complications of high blood pressure and diabetes can be reduced by the delivery of effective healthcare. Crucially, this entails:

- Partnership between patients and health professionals with the knowledge, ability and resources to take appropriate measures over many years.
- Cheap and effective drugs and the implementation of simple treatment protocols, as promoted by WHO and the CVD initiative of the Global Forum for Health Research.

An appropriate policy and strategic framework is essential for such initiatives to be effective on a large scale. Even in the poorest countries people are already seeking healthcare for NCDs in both the public and private sectors, particularly in urban areas. Whatever the balance of priorities between different conditions, existing resources should be used as effectively as possible, Rapid evaluation methods can provide policy-makers with information on the current levels and quality of care and identify the main opportunities for improving health services.

The proper planning and co-ordination of NCD prevention and treatment, whether globally or nationally, requires up-to-date data on risk factor and disease levels – currently missing for much of the world. To address this lack, the WHO Non-Communicable Disease and Mental Health Surveillance section is promoting a standardised approach to enable comparisons across regions and over time, preparing the first ever 'world risk status' report for the major NCDs. This will provide a truly global perspective on the size and nature of the problem.

As this article has shown, NCDs are major health problems even in the world's poorest countries, including those regions where infectious diseases continue to take a huge toll. The NCD burden will grow substantially in low and middle-income countries over the next 10 to 20 years. NCDs will increasingly demand attention and require the right balance between competing priorities for prevention, cure and care. In meeting this challenge, national policy-markers will need to follow the lead of WHO and develop a strategic framework that plans for surveillance, prevention and appropriate health sector reforms.

Bibliography

Books

1. Abdul Aziz: *The Rural Poor, Problems and Prospects,* Ashis Publishing House, New Delhi, 1983.
2. Arora. R.C.: *Industry and Rural Development,* S. Chand and Co Pvt. Ltd. 1978.
3. Alexander. R.J.: *"A Primer to Economic Development,"* the Macmillian and Co. Ltd. London 1962.
4. Barn. P.A. *Political Economy of Growth,* New York, 1962.
5. Behari. Bepin, *Rural Industrialisation in India,* Vikas Publishing House Pvt. Ltd., New Delhi, 1976.
6. Bhattacharya. S.N.: *"Development of Industrial Backward Area" (Indian Style) Metro politan*, Pragati Press, through V.R.N. Composing Agency, Delhi, 1981.
7. Bhojendra Nath Benerjee, *Industry Agriculture and Rural Development.* B.R. Publishing Corporation, New Delhi, 1987.
8. Cykor. G. *Strategies for Industrialisation in Developing Countries,* C. Hurst and Co., London 1974.
9. Dandekar V.M. *Poverty in India,* New Delhi, The Ford Foundation, 55, Lodi House, 1970.
10. Desai Vasanth: *Problems and Prospects Small Scale Industries,* Himalaya Publishing House, Bombay 1983.
11. Eygene Staleey and Richard Morse; *Modern Small Scale Industry for Developing Countries,* Mc Graw Hill Book Co, New York 1965.

10. Sheela Bhide, *Development of Small Scale Industries, Collaborative Approach,* Economic and Political Weekly, December 9, 2000, P. 4389.

11. Dr. Soundara Pandian M. *District Industries Centre for Small Enterprise Development Issues and Solution,* Kurukshetra, December 2000, P. 12.

12. Smt. Vasumdara Raje, *The Role of S.S.I. in Promoting Economic Development,* Southern Economist, Vol. 39, Number 4, June 15, 2000, P. 11.

13. Smt. Vasundara Raje (Minister of State Independent Charge) small scale industries Agro & Rural Industries *Government of India, Taking S.S.I. Towards New Millennium Message of Hope,* Laghu Udhyog Samachar April-September 2000 Cover Story.

14. Valasamma Antony. M.S. *"Quarterly Economic Report, The Indian Institute of Public Opinion New Delhi,* Vol. 43, Number 4, October-December 2000, P. 172.

15. Umat. R.C. *The New Industrial and Investment Policy,* Yojana, July 16-31, 1991, P. 8.

Reports

Industrial Potential Survey Report of Kurnool District, Report Prepared by Commissioner of Industries, Hyderabad.

Government of Andhra Pradesh, *Statistical Abstract of Andhra Pradesh, Hyderabad,* Directorate of Economics & Statistics 1999-2000.

District Planning Office: *The Hand Book of Statistics Kurnool District,* Kurnool 1994-95.

Government of India, First Five Year Plan, Second Five Year Plan, Third Five Year Plan, Annual Plans, Fourth Five Year Plan, Fifth Five Year Plan, Sixth Five Year Plan, Seventh Five Year Plan, Eighth Five Year Plan and Ninth Five Year Plan.

Index

T

U

W